Sex Pos.
Couples

Explore a new sex life experience to boost your couple libido, improve your intimacy and satisfy the desire in your relationship.

Madison Hunter

Table of Contents

Introduction

You might have already heard about this legendary collection of texts in pop culture. Images depicting sensual acts between consenting adults may come into mind at the mere mention of the name. In fact, several movies have already been made based on the teachings in this scripture. It might have been thrown around as a joke or two in some scenes but the term Kama Sutra has become quite synonymous to the amorous affair of making love.

Closely related to matters behind locked bedrooms, this literary piece was compiled by a sage called Vatsyayana Mallanaga for a Hindu audience.

In truth, it is impossible to pinpoint who created these writings, but the modern world is lucky that efforts have been made not just to compile them, but to translate them from ancient Sanskrit to more modern tongues.

For beginners, Hinduism is known as one of the largest religious movements in the world; third largest to be exact. Most of the people who practice Hinduism are from Nepal, India, Bali and Bangladesh.

On top of being one of the largest collections of followers in the world, it is also one of the oldest. It can be said that Hinduism stems from Vedic traditions which hail from a time wherein India had barely discovered iron and have begun utilizing it.

The Vedic tradition is known as the oldest form of worship in the Hindu world and modern Hinduism is based on its teachings. It is surprising to see that a collection of knowledge so old would still have bearings in today's society.

Interestingly, this compilation (The Kama Sutra) isn't just about elaborate measures of coital pleasure. This collection mainly talks about the regular Joe (in ancient Indian times) and how he should live his life amongst the people. It paints pictures of the modern man's life (at that time). From tending to his personal business to nights out with friends and lovers, it covers almost every aspect of a grown Indian man's life.

Not only does it talk about men. It also talks about how women should behave during those times. Think of it as a manual for day-to-day discourse and engaging members of the opposite sex.

It even contains advice on how to attract women.

When you first start having sex, it can seem a bit intimidating. This will include positions that you can try while laying down, sitting, standing, and kneeling. It should give you a good basis to get started on you can continue to branch out from there.

It is important to understand that while some positions may be great for you your partner may not love them. So, trying different things and having an Arsenal of different sex positions to try is advantageous in having excellent sexual sessions. Here again, you need to be open to experimentation. Trying out different positions can lead you to a whole new world of ecstasy that you have never experienced.

Let's start out by looking at some of the most basic sex positions that can be accomplished while laying down and how to actually make them happen. However, they may surprise you once you actually give them a try. So, don't feel as if the basics aren't good enough as often times they absolutely are.

The first position that we would like to look at is the face to face position. To accomplish this both parties will be laying on their sides. You'll be facing each other. The female will be slightly higher on the bed than her male counterpart. This is so that her hips are above his. One of her legs will wrap around the top of him and the other one should be laid down straight. Sometimes this can feel a bit awkward but with practice, it feels truly great.

This is a fantastic position for beginners because it helps you to gain comfort with your partner. It is a very intimate position that will allow deeper levels of penetration. The closeness of this position also helps both to relax and enjoy the experience.

Next, we have one of the most common positions, missionary style. This is done by the female lying flat on her back and the male on top of her. The female's legs can be in a variety of different positions.

Sometimes, she will lay them down flat on the bed while other times she may wrap them around her partner's waist. This simply comes down to what is most comfortable. Other people prefer to have their knees bent so that their feet are flat on the bed and their knees are facing the ceiling.

Missionary position is basic but essential for beginners. It is one of our go-to moves. It allows for different positioning which can help both parties achieve orgasm more easily. It tends to be very comfortable for both the man and the woman. You will be facing each other, and this will allow you to focus on the level of intimacy that you are exuding. Additionally, it will make it easy to communicate what your needs are if the position needs to change slightly.

Chapter 1

Meaning About the Name Kama Sutra

The word Kama is one that means pleasure but can also be translated as desire or longing. There is a sexual connotation associated with the word, meaning it is more to do with sexual pleasure and desire than with the pleasures of life or desire for material goods, but that doesn't mean that the Kama Sutra as a whole is limited to only sexual pleasure. Sutra, on the other hand, translates to verse or scripture. When you put these words together, you get the translation of "Scripture of Pleasure", but there are many variations on how you can literally translate this.

Delving deeper into the meaning behind the name, the pleasure that is Kama is one that is of all five senses, and this is very important.

We know that the Kama Sutra extends beyond just the physical pleasures, now here are four different virtues of life. Those four are:

- Dharma – How to live a virtuous life

- Kama – How to enjoy the pleasures of the senses

- Moksha – How to be liberated from the cycle of reincarnation

- Artha – How to gain material wealth

These four virtues are tenants of Hinduism, which is applicable since the Kama Sutra originates in India where Hinduism is one of the predominant religions. The author saw sexual pleasure as one of the main virtues of life, and it was both a necessary and spiritual pursuit that was important both from a non-sexual and sexual avenue. These virtues are almost instructions on how a person should live in order to be fulfilled both in this life as well as in the afterlife. Regardless of what your personal religion is, all the points are still applicable, as basic human nature dictates that we are all attempting to be the best version of ourselves and to accomplish everything we set out to gain.

Some other words that you may encounter within the Kama Sutra, and their translations, are:

- Devi – Goddess

- Gandharva – A form of marriage in which everyone is consenting to it

- Lingam – Penis

- Nayika – A woman who is desired by someone

- Prahanana – Striking or slapping someone during sex

- Raja – King

- Shlokas – Messages from above that are used to end every topic of the Kama Sutra

- Vatsala – A married woman who has children

- Vikrant – A brave and beloved man

- Yoni – Vagina

So why does the literal meaning of the name even matter?

If you come into the Kama Sutra thinking it should only include some sex positions and nothing more, then you miss out on the richness that is contained within. Likewise, if you ignore the historical significance behind the text, you fail to grasp many of the concepts located within. In order to gain as much as you can from the Kama Sutra, you need to know what the author intended with it, and why they felt the need to create this work of literature.

History of the Kama Sutra

The exact date that the Kama Sutra was written is not known, but estimates place it anywhere between 400 BCE and 300 CE. What we do know, however, is that it was officially and we know today in the 2nd century, otherwise known as 2 CE. This does not mean though that it has not undergone revisions since then, and some scholars believe that the version we have is actually closely linked to the 3rd century, as some of the references throughout would not have been applicable to the 2nd century. With the text being so old, exact dating is virtually impossible, nevertheless, there is a lot of information we do know about it.

We do know that the text originates from India, although the exact location is unknown. Historians have been able to narrow down the location to somewhere within the north, or northwest, region but beyond that, it is a guess as to where the author was from.

Since it's compilation in the 2nd-3rd century, it has undergone numerous translations and there are versions in almost every language. It was originally written in Sanskrit, an ancient Indian language, and this is the language that many Hindu scriptures were written in. While some translations are quite accurate, it is important to note that some translators did place their own bias into their work and that can be seen in the discrepancies that were found. One of the key examples of this was in the 19th century, when the Kama Sutra was translated into English. The translator at that time wanted to ensure that the role of women in the sexual realm was not as prominent, as that was not the culture of the times. In order to maintain that societal understanding of sex and women, the Kama Sutra was altered so that women were significantly downplayed throughout. This has since been corrected, but it is important to be aware of this if you ever decide to pick up a copy for yourself as you want to be sure you are getting a purer translation.

The foundations are rooted within the Vedic Era of literature, which is based on the word Vedas. Vedas were historical texts written in India around this time that dealt with lifestyle and how one should conduct themselves on a daily basis. All works of this time period were verbally passed down, and traditions were adapted into many of the Hindu beliefs that are now practiced today. In the Vedic Era, there were distinct classes and castes within society, and a lot of that is reflected within the Kama Sutra. Many references are made to those who are in differing classes, and how relationships between individuals of different castes cannot work out. While this type of information is not apparently meaningful in today's culture, it does cross over when we look at socio-economic statuses and how the rich and poor interact even today.

Philosophy of the Kama Sutra

As we said, we do know a bit about why Vatsyayana wrote the Kama Sutra. Many of the texts focused on the two important virtues of Dharma (morality), and Athra (prosperity), while few really delved into the importance of Kama (pleasure). Vatsyayana meditated upon this reality and came to the conclusion that Kama was just as important as all of the other virtues, and so it was only proper to have a guide written solely about how to obtain Kama.

The four virtues can be looked at more as goals that each person much work towards within their lifetime in order to lead a complete and fulfilled life. Within the Kama Sutra, there are many references to the other virtues as they are all tied together and must be achieved in order to succeed. One cannot simply focus on the physical pleasures and ignore the need for morality or prosperity, so you may notice throughout that sex and morality are often combined, as well as sex and finding a partner that brings about monetary prosperity.

To understand the philosophy behind the Kama Sutra, it is vital that you understand what it was intended to be. The sex acts that are described throughout are little more than theatrics, with an emphasis on outrageous and yoga-inspired poses. The goal was unlikely to be used as a literal manual, but instead to be used as a way to understand both society and the individual. It can be seen as almost a screenplay, taking us on a journey of love within ancient Indian times. There is talk of love, intimacy, and mundane tasks such as bathing and grooming. The Kama Sutra is a manual on all aspects of pleasure, both in the sexual sense and in the day to day realm.

Kama is so often seen as something that is less important than other aspects of human pursuit. We are told to work hard, earn money, find a spouse, have children, and live a moral and righteous life. But rarely are advised on how to let loose and enjoy ourselves, or how important of a role sex plays in the human experience. The Kama Sutra is the bridge over that gap, intended to lift up the importance of pleasure and sex, and place it in as high of regard as all the other aspects we are expected to work towards.

Chapter 2

How to use Kama Sutra

Kama Sutra is the oldest in the world love treatise written by the Indian sage Mallanaga Vatsyayana, who lived in the III-IV century BC. The Kama Sutra has a collection of all the ancient Indian erotic concepts, knowledge and wisdom accumulated from thousands of amorous couples for centuries. In ancient India, it was decided to give leadership, like the at Kama Sutra, to the girls who were approaching the stage of puberty. It was done to help them to discover their sexuality and to accelerate the development of femininity.

Assuming that Kama Sutra is a description of several thousand of sexual positions and techniques, it is wrong. There is another misconception. Many believe that most of the methods described in the Kama Sutra are so complicated that they can be practiced only by a very well-trained and physically developed people. While in fact, you do not need to have any exceptional strength or acrobatic training to use the Indian's knowledge into practice.

Most of these errors are related to the fact that the West still does not exist in the counterpart of Kama Sutra. The vast majority of Western publications on the subject - it's either outright pornography or medical references, so oversaturated with anatomical details that reading them is enough for a person to stop treating sex as high art permanently. But in fact, many of us tend to view sex as just a means of procreation, or as an opportunity to meet the low-lying physiological instinct.

In contrast, the sexual act in the East initially was considered a sacred ritual, and the relationship between men and women consistently described in highly artistic, poetic form. This is the difference between the wealthiest language of love of the East and our own. Yes, to begin with, the fact that in our language so far, there are no adequate words to refer to reproductive organs. Only so challenging to pronoun Kama Sutra is the oldest in the world love treatise written by the Indian sage Mallanaga Vatsyayana, who lived in the III-IV century BC. The Kama Sutra has a collection of all the ancient Indian erotic concepts, knowledge and wisdom accumulated from thousands of amorous couples for centuries. In ancient India, it was decided to give leadership, like Kama Sutra, to the girls who were approaching the stage of puberty. It was done to help them to discover their sexuality and to accelerate the development of femininity.

Today the Kama Sutra - without a doubt, is famous in the world pertaining to erotica. Assuming that Kama Sutra is a description of several thousand of sexual positions and techniques, it is wrong. There is another misconception. Many believe that most of the methods described in the Kama Sutra are so complicated that they can be practiced only by a very well-trained and physically developed people. While in fact, you do not need to have any exceptional strength or acrobatic training to use the Indian's knowledge into practice.

"No one knows the boundaries of the possible love of women, even those to whom she gives her tenderness because the woman's love has a special delicacy. Men rarely learn the women in their right light, also though they may love them or be indifferent to them, to admire them or leave them, even when they try to learn from all the women than the ones possess." The Kama Sutra

Thus, here we find the exact opposite of the image of women that are prevalent in men in the West. The Kama Sutra is not about how a woman occupies a subordinate position, playing the role of a "passive bottom." The woman has an active, creative side, and it may well take a lead role in a love match. Kama Sutra affirms the equality of both sexes, the absolute equality of men and women. Neither sex dominates, does not assert its supremacy, and the dominant position may occupy a man or a woman alternately. None of the partners cannot and should not take more than what they are capable of giving. At the heart of all the sexual techniques described in the Kama Sutra, it is unselfish mutual love. And between the two of the loving people, there is no place for selfish desire to possess. It is imperative to understand all those who seek to find true freedom in sex and to experience the fullness of its actual existence.

To be successful in love, each person must continuously improve. The Kama Sutra lists the sixty-four arts, which are recommended to study on par with the art of love. It includes; singing, music, poetry, painting, logical exercises, learning foreign languages, housekeeping, cooking, sports and martial arts. The art of beautiful dressing and even acting. Mastery of these skills helps a person become more harmonious, allows learning much more sensitively and subtly perceives the world around us and helps us see the beauty of the human body. Secondly, having all of these arts, a man with great ease will be able to locate and attract anyone and be educated, elegant, and much more attractive in the eyes of the opposite sex.

We now turn to another critical aspect. In the Kama Sutra, as well as in other ancient Eastern teachings about love, the physical body is a temple of our soul, the microcosm of our universe. In the old Oriental mystical philosophical concept, known as Tantra, there is the idea that no temple is built by humans, it does not exceed the holy temple of the human body. In the human anatomy there is a place where all the elements of life; ether, air, fire, water, and earth are found. According to Tantra, God is our higher self, or our soul, which we serve through our body temple.

In the bodily temple, there are nine "gates," upper and lower. The lower gates are the genitals and anus. High barriers are the mouth, nose, ears, and fontanel on the crown of the head. According to the Eastern Esoteric concepts through the fontanel, called Hole of Brahma, the immortal soul at birth enters the body temple and, after death, leaves it.

The act of servicing the body temple is the concentration of sexual energy. Ecstatic enlightenment process begins at the site of the genital's location, and then the sacred fire of love gradually fills the entire human body, burning all the negative energy and illuminating the temple of the body. Thus, having sex is perceived by followers of Tantra as a kind of rite designed to purify the human body from all sin and evil, and bring it true freedom. It is crucial to treat your own body as a temple, and not as something shameful, "unclean" and a sinful thing to hide in the darkness, not only from the eyes of strangers but from the eyes of a loved one. Our body, the temple, must be kept clean and healthy out of respect for the divine that lies within our own physical body. No need to spare any non-effort to ensure that the full delight is the divine within. No need to hold back and to hide any expression of his passion, so that the present service is a spontaneous and all-consuming act of love.

"No one knows the boundaries of the possible love of women, even those to whom she gives her tenderness because the woman's love has a special delicacy. Men rarely learn the women in their right light, also though they may love them or be indifferent to them, to admire them or leave them, even when they try to learn from all the women than the ones possess." The Kama Sutra

Thus, here we find the exact opposite of the image of women that are prevalent in men in the West. The Kama Sutra is not about how a woman occupies a subordinate position, playing the role of a "passive bottom." The woman has an active, creative side, and it may well take a lead role in a love match. Kama Sutra affirms the equality of both sexes, the absolute equality of men and women. Neither sex dominates, does not assert its supremacy, and the dominant position may occupy a man or a woman alternately. None of the partners cannot and should not take more than what they are capable of giving. At the heart of all the sexual techniques described in the Kama Sutra, it is unselfish mutual love. And between the two of the loving people, there is no place for selfish desire to possess. It is imperative to understand all those who seek to find true freedom in sex and to experience the fullness of its actual existence.

.

Chapter 3

What Kama sutra says about love?

When it comes to love, there is much that can be said on how to obtain it, maintain it, and nourish it. While sex and love do not always go hand in hand, the Kama Sutra does emphasize the importance of love and goes to great lengths in order to detail exactly how a person can find love and then how they should go about ensuring that it lasts for a lifetime. Love begins with oneself, and only then can it be extended beyond that and onto someone else. That is why the Kama Sutra makes sure to include ways to enhance your own inner love and desire but focusing on self-care and self-adornment. The more you love yourself the more you can love others, and the more they can love you in return. If you are down on yourself, lack self-worth, or generally feel unlovable, then you will project that onto everyone that you come in contact with. You need to be able to present the best version of yourself possible, and always remember, there is nothing sexier in life than confidence!

Love is an extremely complex concept, and while we all may feel we understand what love is, if you ask 100 individuals to define love you will end up with 100 different responses. Love is defined as the feeling of attraction and desire that one feels towards another, but if you have ever been in love you will know that it extends far beyond that shallow explanation. Love and lust can often be confused with one another, since both play on attraction and desire, but the simplest way to break the two apart is to see love as something that is long-term, whereas lust oftentimes will fade or develop into love. When it comes to love, there are many factors that go into both falling in love, as well as staying in love with someone. Love is not easy, nor is it free from work, and in order to maintain a healthy, loving relationship you must be willing to sacrifice, compromise, and put in effort daily. Love is something that can grow and deepen with time, like a tree grows its roots down into the earth. What begins as only a small sapling can eventually turn into a mighty oak that even the worst of storms cannot damage. But how does one grow that tree of love? And how does one nurture it so that it is not cut down with time?

The understanding of this concept has never really been clear to mankind for if that had been the case then marital lives of many would be very different from what they are today. We can't simply blame the present rise in divorce rates in the current generation or on love marriages, for our understanding of a successful marriage is very narrow, and accepting one where the couple stays together till one of them dies. But a marriage or a relationship where you have felt like a captive is not a happy union at all. While we sure can't change the mentality of the masses regarding arranged marriages, or simply marriages, what we can do is ensure that we find the right person to love, and that isn't as simple as finding someone who loves you as much as you love him.

When you are beginning to make love for the first number of times, you may feel awkward, wondering what positions you should do or what the other person may prefer. You may feel pressure to perform or to please your partner better than they've ever been pleased before. All of these thoughts are normal, but it is rare that a person will be an expert the first time or even the first ten times they do something new. The great thing about sex, though, is that it is a natural act for humans to engage in, which means there will be some amount of innate knowledge you will have about how to conduct yourself in a sexual encounter. Keeping that in mind, you will need to be able to trust yourself and your body in order to make the most of your first several sexual experiences.

There are some things that you must be aware of when it comes time for your first sexual encounter. Following the point that was just made above, the first thing to know is to trust yourself! At the most basic level, humans are animals. Just like any other animal, we are meant to have sex. This means that sex comes wired into our DNA and that we all have some knowledge of how to conduct ourselves during sexual intercourse. This is because our body is able to take over and follow its pleasure, its arousal and its instincts. While you don't want to act like a complete animal in bed (unless you and your partner are into it), this is simply useful to keep in mind so that you can keep your nerves at bay. If you let your mind take control, it will get in the way of and inhibit this natural instinct that you came built with.

This leads us to the next things to know, which is that relaxation and being at ease will make the encounter much more enjoyable for both of you. If you are able to relax and enjoy the experience, your body will flow much smoother, and pleasure will come much easier to both you and your partner.

Chapter 4

Tantric Sex

Tantra is a mystical philosophical, psychological and cosmological concept.

Tantra doctrine found expression in numerous Tantric writings, works of art, in alchemical experiments, and magic rituals.

The aim of the followers of Tantric teachings is reconciliation and merging of the existing in the world of opposites. Tantra rejects the carnal, bodily side of life. Tantra accepts the man as he is, with all his feelings, desires, natural needs, and instincts.

The central concept of Tantra is Reality (ultimate reality, understood as a single, indivisible whole). The truth in the Indian language is called Shiva-Shakti. This name is deriving from the name of the supreme God in the Hindu- Lord Shiva and Goddess Shakti, that is supreme. Each person can comprehend the higher reality and identify with Shiva and Shakti, the original space of the loving couple. All earthly love couples are just like these supreme couples.

Tantra cannot be called a religion in the strict sense of the word.

Most Tantra's are a set of practices that help to enhance human abilities, and especially of human consciousness. The word Tantra derives from the Sanskrit root "tan", which means expanding. Experimental methods of Tantra have nothing to do with the empty verbiage and meaningless chatter. Tantric teachers have developed several specific, empowering social practices; breathing and gymnastic exercises, meditation techniques, and powerful repetition of sounds and phrases (mantras), and, finally, sexual techniques. The latter is not surprising, because it allows performing a sexual act to reconcile the two most pronounced opposites - male and female. And it more than meets the main task of Tantra teachings. The sexual act refers to the whole group of those rituals that must be performed in a specific order. Implementation of these practices will lead to the fact that all the contradictions in the minds of the Tantra adept merge, and they can thereby escape from the endless cycle of rebirth, physical, and spiritual development.

Tantric sex - Sexual interaction of men and women in the tradition of Tantra - it is something more than just sex. Tantric sexual practices were created to transform human sexual energy into the power of spiritual liberation. With the help of these sexual practices, a couple can identify with the primordial forces of nature and learn to manage them. Through this approach to sexuality, each pair can grasp the hidden, deeper meaning of lovemaking, the sense that is available only to the elite.

It looks fantastic by the fact that many Tantric practices were found among the Australian Aborigines, the representatives of the indigenous population that is so far from the Indian continent. However, a closer consideration of similarity in the practices of the Australian Aborigines and the adepts of Tantra does not seem unlikely. Australian Aborigines are close to Indian tribal peoples. Their languages are similar.

Tantra in the West is perceived as a "sex religion." This attitude is based on the fact that Tantra's followers did not see any sense to fight with their natural sensual drives and preaching, free from all sorts of prohibitions outlook on life. One of the basic principles of Tantra's teachings is that any suppression of our nature violates our inner harmony. All of the body's emotional and mental commitment must be focused on this setting, although it may seem like pandering own faults and weaknesses. However, self-indulgence rarely becomes the result of the natural tendency.

In contrast, self-indulgence comes from a lack of emotional and psychological maturity. For a man, it is imperative to learn to distinguish natural from unnatural desires. This view is a unique feature of the Tantric tradition. All other religious and philosophical teachings prescribe their followers the need to suppress such desires as hunger, the need for sleep and sex drive. Tantra teaches that the suppression of natural attractions can cause significant harm to both physical and psychological health, causing severe neurosis or mental illness. Although the destruction of natural desires may temporarily lead to the desired effect, for an extended period, it causes great harm. Very rarely, actual spiritual development can be achieved, employing repression and prohibition.

A Tibetan story that tells about a man named Sarvabhaksha, who survived until our era. He was suffering from binge eating; he was obsessive and had an utterly irresistible desire to devour everything edible that fell into his hands. Once Sarvabhaksha met a Tantric guru Saraha and asked him for advice about how to deal with this problem. The guru had taught him to imagine his stomach empty as clear sky, and the hunger and the desire for the absorption of food - a fire that will consume him and the world around him. Tantra's teacher advised Sarvabhaksha to imagine that during the meal, he devoured the entire universe. Finally, the guru told him to believe that all things and phenomena of the world are non-existent, which causes nothing but emptiness behind them.

Chapter 5

Differences between Kama sutra sex and Tantric sex

Kama Sutra is the oldest in the world love treatise written by the Indian sage Mallanaga Vatsyayana, who lived in the III-IV century BC. The Kama Sutra has a collection of all the ancient Indian erotic concepts, knowledge and wisdom accumulated from thousands of amorous couples for centuries. In ancient India, it was decided to give leadership, like the Kama Sutra, to the girls who were approaching the stage of puberty. It was done to help them to discover their sexuality and to accelerate the development of femininity.

Penned in what is considered to be a highly sophisticated form of the Sanskrit language, the title of what we now know as the Kama Sutra means – "a treatise on pleasure". This refers to all the pleasures of life, from eating and drinking to that greatest of all pleasures – sex. But it also refers to the intellectual pleasures of life and how these contribute to sexual happiness. The Kama Sutra is very unique for a text of this time period, as it's geared to the enlightenment of both men and women and, as such, was probably the very first work of literature intended to be enjoyed equally by both sexes.

"Pleasure" in the Kama Sutra's terms, is a holistic concept that encompasses all facets of life. It's most compelling mission is to teach people to get the most out of life by enjoying it in the moment and as a joyful adventure. Particularly geared to teaching its readers and adherents how to go about getting the most from their romantic partnerships, the Kama Sutra sees that project as a combination of many things, all working together to create a harmonious life that plays out in harmonious relationships.

For the Kama Sutra, relationships are a type of performance art, performed in the theatre of life. They are not divorced from it, as private worlds. Unfortunately, the West tends to divorce couples in an odd sort of way, with many people retreating into a world in which friends must also be coupled in order for friendships to survive. But society is the couple's context and so the Kama Sutra provides detailed information about how society works and where romantically-linked couples fit into it and participate in it. This includes how one goes about finding a partner, for both men and women.

Now let's talk about Tantric Sex. Tantra is a mystical philosophical, psychological and cosmological concept.

Tantra doctrine found expression in numerous Tantric writings, works of art, in alchemical experiments, and magic rituals.

The aim of the followers of Tantric teachings is reconciliation and merging of the existing in the world of opposites. Tantra rejects the carnal, bodily side of life. Tantra accepts the man as he is, with all his feelings, desires, natural needs, and instincts.

The central concept of Tantra is Reality (ultimate reality, understood as a single, indivisible whole). The truth in the Indian language is called Shiva-Shakti. This name is deriving from the name of the supreme God in the Hindu- Lord Shiva and Goddess Shakti, that is supreme. Each person can comprehend the higher reality and identify with Shiva and Shakti, the original space of the loving couple. All earthly love couples are just like these supreme couples.

Tantra cannot be called a religion in the strict sense of the word.

Most Tantra's are a set of practices that help to enhance human abilities, and especially of human consciousness. The word Tantra derives from the Sanskrit root "tan", which means expanding. Experimental methods of Tantra have nothing to do with the empty verbiage and meaningless chatter. Tantric teachers have developed several specific, empowering social practices; breathing and gymnastic exercises, meditation techniques, and powerful repetition of sounds and phrases (mantras), and, finally, sexual techniques. The latter is not surprising, because it allows performing a sexual act to reconcile the two most pronounced opposites - male and female. And it more than meets the main task of Tantra teachings. The sexual act refers to the whole group of those rituals that must be performed in a specific order. Implementation of these practices will lead to the fact that all the contradictions in the minds of the Tantra adept merge, and they can thereby escape from the endless cycle of rebirth, physical, and spiritual development.

Tantric sex - is not just postures and techniques described in any modern textbook of love. Sexual interaction of men and women in the tradition of Tantra - it is something more than just sex. Tantric sexual practices were created to transform human sexual energy into the power of spiritual liberation. With the help of these sexual practices, a couple can identify with the primordial forces of nature and learn to manage them. Through this approach to sexuality, each pair can grasp the hidden, deeper meaning of lovemaking, the sense that is available only to the elite.

It looks fantastic by the fact that many Tantric practices were found among the Australian Aborigines, the representatives of the indigenous population that is so far from the Indian continent. However, a closer consideration of similarity in the practices of the Australian Aborigines and the adepts of Tantra does not seem unlikely. Australian Aborigines are close to Indian tribal peoples. Their languages are similar.

Tantra in the West is perceived as a "sex religion." This attitude is based on the fact that Tantra's followers did not see any sense to fight with their natural sensual drives and preaching, free from all sorts of prohibitions outlook on life. One of the basic principles of Tantra's teachings is that any suppression of our nature violates our inner harmony. All of the body's emotional and mental commitment must be focused on this setting, although it may seem like pandering own faults and weaknesses. However, self-indulgence rarely becomes the result of the natural tendency.

Chapter 6

Physical Attraction of Love

Physical Attraction and Love

Although love requires much more than a simple physical attraction, the way a person looks is oftentimes the first thing that draws us to them. When you are looking to meet someone, and you know nothing about them as a person, you are going solely off of how they look to you. If someone is physically unattractive in your eyes, there is very little chance that you will want to pursue something intimate with them and thus the road to love is cut short.

We are in no way suggesting that your appearance is the only thing about you that matters, but we are saying that you should pamper and care for yourself in order to be the best version of yourself that you can be. From good hygiene practices to wearing your favorite sexy dress, making yourself look good will also make you feel good and that creates an energy that will draw someone to you.

When you are beginning to make love for the first number of times, you may feel awkward, wondering what positions you should do or what the other person may prefer. You may feel pressure to perform or to please your partner better than they've ever been pleased before. All of these thoughts are normal, but it is rare that a person will be an expert the first time or even the first ten times they do something new. The great thing about sex, though, is that it is a natural act for humans to engage in, which means there will be some amount of innate knowledge you will have about how to conduct yourself in a sexual encounter. Keeping that in mind, you will need to be able to trust yourself and your body in order to make the most of your first several sexual experiences.

Things to Know for Your First Time

There are some things that you must be aware of when it comes time for your first sexual encounter. Following the point that was just made above, the first thing to know is to trust yourself! At the most basic level, humans are animals. Just like any other animal, we are meant to have sex. This means that sex comes wired into our DNA and that we all have some knowledge of how to conduct ourselves during sexual intercourse. This is because our body is able to take over and follow its pleasure, its arousal and its instincts. While you don't want to act like a complete animal in bed (unless you and your partner are into it), this is simply useful to keep in mind so that you can keep your nerves at bay. If you let your mind take control, it will get in the way of and inhibit this natural instinct that you came built with.

This leads us to the next things to know, which is that relaxation and being at ease will make the encounter much more enjoyable for both of you. If you are able to relax and enjoy the experience, your body will flow much smoother, and pleasure will come much easier to both you and your partner.

The next thing to note is the importance of foreplay. In case you are unsure, foreplay is any and all of the sexual activities that come before the actual act of sexual intercourse. This can include the making out and groping, the handjob or fingering as well as oral sex or anything else you engage in before penetration occurs. This part of sex is just as important as the rest of sex because this is when you become aroused and let your arousal build before beginning penetration. It is during this time that you are able to explore each other's bodies and figure out where the other person likes to be touched the most.

Communication is the final thing to note for the first time. It may seem like there is an expectation to pretend like you know exactly what you are doing and that you have done it a thousand times before, but this is untrue. No matter who your partner is, they will be happy that you communicated and made sure that they were comfortable all along the way instead of pretending like you knew exactly what they wanted. Being able to communicate in bed is more impressive than not saying anything and guessing the entire time.

We will now look at the best sex positions for your first time. With so many possible sex positions to do, it can be overwhelming trying to decide which ones to try first. I will explain and describe the best positions for you to use during your first several sexual encounters. Keep in mind as well, that many people continue to have sex in these positions well after their first time, simply because they find the most pleasure from these positions. These are by no means reserved for your first couple of sexual encounters, especially if you thoroughly enjoy them.

Chapter 7

Different Type of Love

The Kama Sutra breaks down three different types of love, which are:

- Continual Habit

- Imagination

- Belief

These three types of love are not necessarily limited to just within a relationship, and they can be extended to other aspects of life as well. Below will we break down these different forms of love, how they relate to your personal love life, and even give advice on how to create, maintain, and nourish each type.

Love by Habits

Love by continual habit is described in the Kama Sutra as the love that comes from repetition and practice of an act. In a non-romantic way, this is the love that may develop for a certain hobby as you continue to practice it and get better at it. The more you engage yourself and learn, the more you develop a love and passion. In a romantic way, this is the love that develops over long periods of time with an individual, either within or outside of a romantic relationship. For example, some people may begin as friends long before they become lovers. Over time, as they do activities together, engage in long, deep talks, and grow as people they eventually fall in love. This is the continual habit of being around someone and continuing to learn about them and grow together as a couple. This is a very strong form of love, as there is a great foundation to it, and it is built not on lust but completely on love.

This is also part of what forms the love between two individuals who have been together for many years. Over the years that initial sexual attraction may begin to fade, and the lust that drew you together will start to become more of a slow-burning flame that keeps you both going. It is at this point that continual habit starts to strengthen and create the love between two people, as you live together and work together you practice the art of being in love. Falling in love is not the end, it is only the beginning, and over the years you will need to continuously work on that love and nurture it so that it continues to grow. Like blowing life into a fire, you are responsible for ensuring that the flame does not burn out.

Love by continual habit should also be extended to the individual, separate from any type of relationship. You should continuously work on learning to love yourself, showering yourself with affection, and strengthening those emotions within yourself. Make yourself into the partner that you so desire, so that whether or not you find that person, you already know you have that completely on your own. If you can meet your own needs, satisfy yourself, and be happy when alone, then a partner is simply the icing on the cake instead of the entire cake itself.

So, how do you create, maintain, and nourish love by continual habit?

• Actively spend time with the person you love or want to be in love with

• Practice being emotionally vulnerable with your partner

• Frequently touch your partner each day

• Take time each day to look in the mirror and appreciate something about yourself

• Share and create memories together

• Develop an idea of the future that you both would like to work towards

• Engage in sex frequently

These are only a very few of the ways in which you can create love via continual habit, and how you choose to do so is a completely personal choice. What is important is not how you do it, but more so doing it in a way that creates happiness and joy in both you and your partner. It is about building and growing together and working at love every day through the practice of making it into a habit.

Love by Imagination

Love by imagination is in complete contrast to love by continual habit, as it is far from physical and exists purely within the mind. This is the type of love that has no bearing in the real world, and instead is created within a fantasy of your choosing. An innate type of love, it is one that already exists within you and requires no effort or forming of habits in order to induce. It is a type of love that exists before your partner and will continue to exist despite your partner as it is not created by them. It can, however, be influenced and informed by your partner, but for the most part, it is simply an innate feeling that you have.

To break this down in more practical terms, we can start by looking at this love in non-romantic ways. Love by imagination is the way you love scary movies, or your love for dogs over cats. It's your love for sweet treats, spicy foods, or taking walks in nature. It's the love you feel when you think about your favorite book or movie, or when you ponder your future and all the things you will accomplish. As you can see, this type of love requires no effort and does not exist because you have worked on it. Instead, it is a love that is easy, effortless, and oftentimes cannot be changed. You can, however, alter this type of love as you age and grow, and different experiences will shape and guide our love by imagination. When you are young you may hate spicy foods, but as your taste buds mature you then find yourself with a passion for the heat. This requires no effort on your part, however, it does change and grow over time.

In a romantic sense, this is the type of love that exists even before you find your partner. Your personal preference in appearance, your desire for someone funny or smart, your different viewpoints and religions and all those other points that you think of in your head are all part of your imagination. If you close your eyes and visualize your ideal partner, you have love by imagination. Now, this type of love helps guide us towards the correct person for us, but it can also be a hindrance to finding a partner. In some ways, when you fall in love with the idea of someone, you set yourself up for failure. No person is perfect, and there is no one on the planet that will check every box or meet every criteria when it comes to your imaginative person. It is very important that you remember this, as those who seek to find perfection will instead only find loneliness. What you should do is use that love by imagination to guide you towards someone, without the expectation that they will live up to every item on the list. When you use love by imagination to guide you, you go into the relationship with a base of love already there. You know that you love people who have a great sense of humor, so you end up already loving that about your partner. If you know that you love someone who is fiercely intelligent, find a partner who is, and you will truly love that about them.

So, what are some ways in which you can create this type of love and maintain it in the long-term?

• Take the time to get inside your own head and find the qualities that are more important to you

• Always remember that no one is perfect, and find perfection within the imperfections

• Seek out people who match your own morals and standards

- Engage in activities you have a pre-existing love for

- Try out new things to find other activities you love

- Nurture your own interests

- Make meditation a part of your daily routine

Remember, this type of love is innate and is not something you can create over time. Take this as more of a starter love, one which draws you to someone and begins that relationship, rather than something used to maintain it over time. While finding someone with the right qualities will help ensure that you remain attracted long-term, it cannot sustain itself unless you strengthen and deepen that love in other ways as well.

Love from Belief

Love from belief is a love that is understood by both parties and is something felt deep within ourselves. It is the type of love in which we have no questions, no doubts, and no fears. When we truly believe in love, when we believe in our feelings, we know that it is true and real. This is one of the strongest forms of love and it is the one in which meaningful relationships are built upon. Love from belief stems from great communication, high levels of trust, and mutual understanding that you both have developed with time and care. It stems from years of work, as well as effort and actions purposely used to create it.

It can also include the love you feel towards your personal accomplishments or achievements, as well as the love that exists within someone's religious beliefs. When you can feel an unwavering love and devotion, then you know you have love from belief. You are certain and sure of that love, there is no question in your mind that it is real and that you are secure within.

For romantic relationships, this is the love that lasts a lifetime. When you and your partner can look into each other's eyes and see nothing buy love reflected back, then you know that you have love from belief. You both believe to your very core that you love the other person and that they love you in return. You are certain that they have no malicious intent, that their reasons are pure, and that their heartbeats only for you. If you are fully your partners, and they are fully yours, then you are experiencing this form of love and you will feel safe and at home within it. But this love is not without work and effort, and in order to develop it, you need to both prove your trustworthiness, and have it proven to you by your spouse. High levels of communication are required so that you are both on the same page and there are no doubts or questions left between you. Trust must be both created and never broken, for if it is ever to be broken then love by belief will cease to exist.

Some of the ways you can develop this type of love and maintain it are:

• Avoid keeping secrets within a relationship and instead, have an air of transparency

• Talk with your partner daily about both random topics as well as deep, important topics

• Gaze into each other's eyes and feel their love looking back at you

•   Make sex intimate and sensual so that you feel a connection and closeness

•   Allow yourself to be vulnerable with your partner

•   Lean on your partner in times of need, and allow them to lean on you in return

•   Make the effort to cultivate your love by having special date nights

Much of this love stems from a trust within yourself and deep knowledge, so it is important you are in tune with your own feelings and intuitions. It is only by being open to this kind of love that will you ever receive it, and if your heart is closed off then you can never experience love by belief.

Chapter 8

Pre Sex

Seduction

Seduction is the act of persuading someone for sexual arousal and intercourse. It mostly happens through actions and words that tend to attract the attention of the victim. If you wish to become a great seducer, you must orchestrate surprise and avoid familiarity and boredom in your relationship. Notably, surprises influence seduction, and it decreases depending on the surprises you make to your partner. For that reason, you will find relationships fading as a result of the lack of surprises among couples. As too much of surprises could be counterproductive, you should create the best moments to make unexpected moves that please your partner. These surprises have power and take much of the victim's afterthought where they remain glued into it. They build up forms of crystalizing you as a better person. Unfortunately, seduction is gradually becoming a lost art for people who have become so self-centered that we are unable to analyze the outside perspective. The fact that seduction is a social activity it encourages you to pay attention to feedback and put yourself in other people's shoes. This way, you will learn more about your seductive energy and how to express it adequately.

As a result, you will refine your seduction based on the character that best fits you.

Identify your seduction character: Successful seduction depends on how well you understand yourself and the energy you exert toward the victim. The following categories should guide you and create the best seducer out of you.

•   Sirens: They are physically undeniable, highly sexual, and confident. They are perfect in creating sexual awareness which aids in luring their targets.

•   Rakes: They are highly unrestrained and are ready to let go and become enslaved by the love of women.

•   Ideal Lover: They make their targets feel elevated and deserving success. The character makes the target fall in love by bringing the perfect quality out in them.

•   Dandies: They demonstrate the freedom and limited roles in life. Their confident expression of their lifestyle makes their targets imitate and admire them.

•   The Natural: They practice openness and innocence. The value of retaining the impeccable quality makes them admirable and worthy life partners who would be a relief from the world's guilt.

•   Coquettes: They exercise the power of love and desire where they portray themselves as self-sufficient. By denying full access, they increase excitement and value, thus more seduction power

•   Charmers: They are socially friendly and are best in pleasing. The fact that they do not complain or fight influences their seduction.

•   Charismatic: Through their confidence, they create illusions and intense plans that portray them as organized and goal-oriented.

•   The Star: They are ethereal and aim to become an ideal reference when seducing those who are interested in fantasies and dreams. Their appearance makes them identifiable through imaginations.

After analyzing yourself and identifying your category, you will also need to understand your target and maneuvers that will make them surrender. It would be advisable to target those who show a deficiency of your abundance and not try to seduce your type. You should look out for signals of what your target lacks and form the basis of your seduction.

The following are types of seduction targets.

•   Patient Dreamers: They long for exploration and adventure but remain in their boring life.

•   Reformists: They seek to escape custodian sexual life.

•   Virtual Royals: They wish to be treated as special people and live a royal life.

• Prudes: They like to keep things undercover and would not want you to judge them for their actions.

• Dark Stars: They once attracted much attention and would like to regain popularity and adoration.

• Fresher: They consider themselves new to sex life but are ready to explore.

• Conquerors: They need to be met with plans and missions to overcome.

• Exotic Fetishist: They are obsessed with exotics and new experiences.

• Drama lovers: They like to remain fascinated by the happenings and wish to be involved in drama throughout their life.

• The intelligent: They think and analyze everything profoundly and wish to find help in relieving mental barriers.

• The appreciated: Used to be praised and needs someone to focus on other aspects that they can enjoy.

• Aging Toddlers: Portrays immature behavior and needs enabling of the desires and gradually reeling them in.

• Life Savers: They like to act as your savior by making them believe that you need them as a protector; you make them develop an obsession.

• Veterans: Their experience in love and sex life makes them desire to educate others.

• Idol seekers: You must act as an object to provide meaning in life and prompt them to worship you.

• Sensualists: They rely on what their senses command them. You must master and influence their smell, touch, taste, and sight to win them.

Foreplay

Foreplay is an activity at the beginning of a sexual encounter that aims at building sexual arousal and brings orgasm in preparation for sexual intercourse. It is a crucial part of sexual experience and acts as a determinant of satisfaction.

Importance of Foreplay

• Biological: Couples need to indulge in foreplay for it causes erection of both the penis and the clitoris. An erection is crucial for it enhances penetration and orgasm among women. Therefore, it creates the best conditions for biological activity. Besides, foreplay elicits wetness making penetration easier for the couples. Lack of vaginal wetness is associated with painful intercourse and bleeding.

• Psychological: Foreplay is known to instill a feeling of care and security among couples. Failure to make foreplay makes your partner feel neglected and denied emotional assurance. The concern of your partner's feeling before sex serves as an indicator that you are not in for selfish gains but mutual pleasure.

Types of Foreplay

Foreplay is the ultimate time to build tension and sexual chemistry between partners. If you lack mind-blowing sex, you should focus on foreplay. Notably, sex is more realistic and complex than what television and movies show. For that reason, when you intimately touch, smell, hear, and taste your partner, they would argue it as better than penetration.

The following are types of foreplay that you should work before sex.

1. Sexy Materials: You could practice foreplay at any time and manner. You do not have to be naked to engage in foreplay. When at home or work you may watch a sexy movie or read sexy materials. These materials could help you maintain orgasm for hours.

2. Undressing: If you usually take off your clothes before sex, then you might be missing a lot of foreplay. Having your fingers hold your partner's outfits and graze on their body as you undress them is highly stimulating and arousing. Depending on how sensitive they are, you might witness them getting goosebumps.

3. Vagina stroking: It involves how you put your hands down there and caressing on her pants and panties. Light strokes on the region make her wet and stimulated for sex.

4. Kisses and caressing: Though kisses do not lead to sex, most sexual activities involve kisses and touching. As part of foreplay, kisses should start slow and intensify gradually. Kisses on the neck and boobs are most arousing for women.

5.   Boob Action: Teases made on their breasts arouse women. Therefore, you should suck, kiss and rub them, taking advantage of the sensitive nerve ending in the nipples. The foreplay should be done with moderation to avoid hurting your partner.

6.   Dry Hump: It involves gently grinding on your partner. It can happen when naked to show how moody you are. The foreplay plays a significant role in heating the moment for intercourse.

7.   Breathing: Yes, you are right; your breath arouses and stimulates your partner, especially when done on sensitive areas such as genitals and neck. In this case, bad breath would be counterproductive.

8.   Hands-On: Your hands are a piece of efficient equipment when it comes to foreplay. You should use them to grab your partner's breasts, rub their hair, and thighs. In short, use your hands to explore your partner's body unless they say no.

9.   Oral: If you are okay in giving oral, you should incorporate it into your foreplay routine. Be a little bit gentle by teasing, sucking, and licking the clitoris and allowing time.

10. Labia love: As a highly ignored part, labia have numerous nerve endings that are perfect for arousal and stimulation. You can massage them slowly or hold them gently between fingers.

11. Ass: If you and your partner are into stimulation through the anus, then you should try it out effectively. The most ignored nerve endings in the anus cause sexual stimulation, especially if gently licked.

12. Multitask: You may incorporate all of these techniques and concurrently make different moves. With the perfect combination, you make your partner fantasized with enjoyable sexual stimulation

Learning to Make Love

As a couple, you may have similar desires and wants, but the sequence required may differ. In most cases, men are known to take less time to achieve sexual stimulation as compared to women. If you are inexperienced in making love or seem to be unskilled, you need to understand what making love entails. How you approach your partner as well as the way you handle the situation plays a significant role in achieving orgasm. It would be advisable to research what you could be doing wrong if your partner complains of sexual dissatisfaction. Similarly, you could explore additional information on ways to make your lovemaking more lively and enjoyable. The following detailed steps to step guide will help you on how you could be a pro in making love.

1.   Nurture your self-esteem: Appreciating your personality and character is the initial point where you develop an excellent reflection about yourself. You should explore your thoughts honestly and openly to identify the aspect that could be hindering you from attaining your full potential. Similarly, you realize your strengths and weaknesses are making it easier to gauge your potential and select tasks. This way, you will be able to relieve yourself of the things that cannot be changed as well as those that are from the past. Notably, this process requires ample time to internalize the steps you need to take to get rid of negative interactions that always drag you behind. It may even entail adjusting your environment and finding time to do what you enjoy. The critical aspect of improving

your self-esteem is embracing change. As it may be difficult in the initial stage, you need to be patient and perseverant to achieve the benefits of being a confident, healthier, and happier person.

2.   Improve Your Lifestyle: After developing high self-esteem and making the right moves to understand yourself, you remain qualified to build a healthy love life. As you explore those various aspects that will offer guidance on your dating life, you need to keep on developing your confidence and selecting a reasonable target. You will realize that making love involves flirting, teasing, and providing compliments as you aim to take your partner to the bed. Developing your intimacy skills will play a vital role in arousing your mind, which then makes you anticipate a gentle touch and intimacy. Besides, you should note that how you present yourself is an excellent determinant of the partner you win and their perception about you. Therefore, you must get a life and begin to make natural moves of seduction and arousal.

3.   Understand What It Is to Make Love: This is an essential part of making love for you might mistake making love for sex. If you do not see any difference, then you might not have experienced it. Sex is familiar to everyone and involves biomechanical and instinctive intercourse. On the contrary, lovemaking is all about the art of sensual and slow romance. Lovemaking is meant to create a connection between partners. The motivation for lovemaking differs from that of sex. Lovemaking is a complex act of expressing love and satisfying your partner. It is an activity where your body, soul, and mind are equally involved in getting to each other's heart. The openness associated with lovemaking allows all forms of communication, leaving no room for wandering. Lovemaking starts long before intercourse and may continue after that. For that

reason, you should consider lovemaking as an emotional activity but not just undressing and romping on the bed.

4. Pick Perfect Location: Lovemaking should happen in a place where you feel comfortable and undistracted. Therefore, you should ensure that the site you choose for lovemaking is romantic. If you would like to make it more personal, you could select a comfortable room in your house where you are aware of the environment. Be creative while choosing your location and consider aspects such as weather and your partner's preference. Also, the temperature of your preferred location should be in line with the activity ahead as too warm or cold could make it a mess. Remember to put away all forms of distractions to avoid losing the true meaning of making love.

5. Set The Mood: If it is your first time to make love, you need to be sure and comfortable about what you are about to do. Ensure that you are aware of what is about to happen and decide on what outcomes you expect. Similarly, make the ambiance conducive and appropriate for lovemaking. When you are in for it avoid being silly or making tasteless jokes thinking that your partner likes it. Instead, settle on a romantic atmosphere where everything you do aims at soothing them and causing sexual stimulation. With this course, your partner will feel appreciated, safe, and cherished through cuddling and gentle touches. Setting the mood may also involve sexy details such as dirty words, music, movies, dim light, and lingerie. When the attitude is right, you will tell from the responses you get from your partner as well as your body reaction.

6. Focus on Foreplay: It is worth noting that lovemaking starts way before sex hence the importance of engaging in stimulating foreplay. It is the best moment to put off the fears and doubts about

yourself or your partner. Besides, foreplay prepares your bodies for sex, especially when done accordingly. Notably, men may experience different feelings during foreplay, and it is essential to ensure that you please your partner by customizing various forms of foreplay. Most women like it when their partners take time during foreplay and incorporate stimulating touches. You should not be in a hurry or skip foreplay for it is pleasurable and makes your partner submit unconditionally. Ensure you observe your partner's reaction to the different techniques you apply so as not to hurt or annoy them. Making love aims at pleasing your partner as you enjoy too. Be selfless and make them feel pampered, unique, and loved. The selflessness reciprocates, and you should rest assured that it creates a memorable event for both of you.

7.   Pick Positions to Achieve Intimacy: Making love involves openness and finding ways to connect with your partner. The connection can be achieved physically, spiritually, and emotionally. Notably, intimacy is performed depending on the level of contact your body is having with that of your partner. Therefore, you should ensure that your body is in better positions and preferably on face-to-face posture. There are various sex positions that you could apply to please your partner and have the best of experiences in intimacy. Sex positions make it easier to communicate while exploring each other's bodies.

8.   Feedback: Most couples find it hard to share their experiences after sex. It proves challenging for men to provide feedback to women on their performance. However, you should understand that telling each other how you feel could make a significant difference in your intimate life. Besides, this form of communication helps you establish a deep connection. When partners provide positive

feedback, they nurture their confidence towards each other, thus promoting perfection and further exploration. Similarly, correcting each other makes you skillful and well cognitive of your partner's hidden treasures. Lovemaking does not end immediately after sex, and that is why you should continue cuddling after sex to extend intimacy and show appreciation.

Making love is experienced after your mind and body develop feelings and intimate emotions. It is an act that brings you closer to your partner, both emotionally and physically.

How to courtship a man/woman

Courtship is the process by which two people get to know one another and decide if they have the possibility of a future together. Courting is different than dating in that courtship is a bit more serious, often with religious motivations and looking to the future with marriage as the ultimate goal. Sometimes courting can be more restricted than dating – with chaperone supervision, strict physical boundaries, or predetermined periods of interaction. If you want to court a man, you should make sure that you are compatible by spending time together, learning about his interests and background, and talking about your respective goals for the future.

Make your intentions clear. Courtship usually leads to marriage; it is a serious, forward-looking way to determine if you could spend your life with someone.

Be approachable and friendly towards the man you're courting. When you are trying to attract the attention of a man, you should try to make yourself seem as approachable as possible.

Show interest in him. Make it clear that you are interested in courting your man. Send him messages and be responsive when he contacts you.

Get to know his friends. Investing time in building relationships with his friends is a great way to show a man that you are seriously committed to this courtship.

To court a woman into a committed relationship, you need to:

1. Make her feel sexually attracted to you.

In the past, a man would need to mostly focus on showing a woman (and her family) that he was capable of providing for her.

In today's world, most women select men based on how much sexual attraction he makes her feel first. They will take a guy for a "test drive" by having sex with him and trying out a relationship and if it makes her happy, she will stick around.

Many of the women you will meet will not be looking to immediately settle down with a guy and commit to marriage on the first date. Initially, all that most women are interested in is whether or not they feel sexually drawn to you.

After sex has happened and she's got a feel for what a relationship with you seems like, she will then make her decision on how serious she wants to get with you (e.g. just date for a while, be boyfriend and girlfriend for a few years and then break up, get engaged and see how it feels or begin talking about and planning your future together as a married couple).

2. Take things to a sexual level.

When guiding a modern woman through the courtship process, you usually can't waste too much time "dating" without actually having sex.

If you wait too long, a woman may end up going out with her girlfriends and having sex on the first with a guy that she meets in a bar or nightclub. Once they've had sex, the relationship will begin and you will probably be left behind.

If you want the courtship to feel amazing for her, you must include sexual attraction and when it is appropriate, you should move in for a kiss and get to sex.

Women today are open to having sex very quickly. It's not 1900 anymore where a man and a woman had to wait until the wedding night to have sex.

These days, almost all couples have plenty of sex during the courtship process to test each other out and see how they feel.

3. Treat her like a potential wife.

If you are serious about courting a woman into a committed relationship or marriage, you shouldn't treat her like yet another girl that you're dating.

Once you and her have talked about wanting to be serious with each other, you need to get rid of any other that you're dating and treat your chosen woman as the one.

Once you and her have talked about wanting to be serious with each other, you need to get rid of any other that you're dating and treat your chosen woman as the one.

4. Take the relationship to the next level.

After being together for a while, you will either gradually progress through the 5 stages of a relationship and into a marriage, or you won't.

Sometimes, a man and a woman will be against marriage and will instead take things to the next level by moving in together, having children and getting a mortgage together for example.

Whatever it is for you is fine, but if you're serious about courting her into a lifelong relationship, always make sure that you are moving towards higher stages of your relationship and commitment together, rather than getting stuck at a certain point and then eventually getting bored of that type of relationship.

Personally speaking, I eventually decided to accept my girlfriend's marriage proposal because it just seemed like the right thing to do. We got married back in April and I now look at it as one of the best decisions I've ever made in life.

The type of love, respect, attraction and commitment you will have for each other when you get married feels nothing like the experience of being in a dating relationship or a boyfriend/ girlfriend relationship.

Chapter 9

Sex Position

Let me begin by asking you if you had sex positions in your yearly goals. I mean if you are in an intimate relationship, this should be one of the goals. If not, it's never too late!

Importance of sex positions

- You get a different view

During the change of positions, you also get to change the places of accomplices as to one another, accordingly, you change viewpoints, perspectives and snugness of accomplices' bodies. As such: You change the image they see. Also, in its turn, the image impacts the accomplices' view of what is happening and their sentiments. It is particularly significant for men, as their eyes are the subsequent delicate zone after penis on its significance. It does not shock

anyone that ladies love with their ears and men with their eyes!))
Men to a great extent live the sex outwardly, that is the reason they
cherish such a great amount to watch pornography. Hearing, the
feeling of touch and smell of men are additionally initiated during
sex, however, above all, they are energized by the image, that is the
thing that they see. Furthermore, for instance, doggy style places of
the opened female rider, when the man see a brilliant perspective
on lady's rump and when he sees his penis infiltrate into his female
accomplice and makes her shudder of joy.

•   It brings different expressions

To see better the interconnection between all sex positions as
well as the sentiments you got that you have to comprehend
the accompanying things: in each position the penis enters
under various point and with various profundity by invigorating
various pieces of the vagina, its various zones and with various
force. As the inward surface of the vagina is sullied (has diverse
reasonableness), the sentiment of a lady in various positions will be
additionally extraordinary. At that, each lady has her sentiments,
which can contrast from the sentiment of another lady. Men, in
this connection, have nearly a similar circumstance: in various
positions, they have a diverse effect on the leader of their penis, on
its various territories.

The sex bucket list

One of the most beautiful things about sex is the ability to get
experimental and try out new things with your partner. Whether
you're trying a new position or bringing some toys into the
bedroom, there are unlimited possibilities for you and your partner

get off. And thanks to porn, TV, movies, and the Internet, as well as the endless articles and magazine written on one of the world's favorite topics, infinite inspiration for experimentation is always at your disposal.

But when it comes down to it, there are certain things that, without a doubt, you must try at least once in the bedroom (or outdoors). That's why I encourage you to come up with an Ultimate Sex Bucket List to unleash your curious side. Sex in public? Definitely. Sex with more than one person? Of course! Mastering the female orgasm? Oh hell yeah. And beyond the obvious things you've fantasized about, I've included some others for your consideration. You'll never know how much you love food in the bedroom or handcuffing your partner unless you try it.

- Sex in Public

- Threesome

- Add A Toy

- Swinging

- The G-Spot Orgasm

- Sex Marathon

- Sex With Food

Different type of sex Positions

The moment you have been waiting for. Finally, some sex positions to try out. Make sure that you understand that most of these take practice to get down, so do not get discouraged if they do not work the first time. Just try something else and move on. Some positions may be easier than others, and some require a little bit of flexibility.

Of course, sex alone will not save or make a relationship. There is so much more to the ordeal than just sleeping together. You have to show your partner love and care as well, and be there for them emotionally and physically, and they should do the same for you. However, when coupled with attentive lovemaking and varied sex positions, you can keep the passion going for a long time.

Sex positions

Of course, there are few sex positions that everyone knows about, and has probably been done. There is missionary, "Doggy style" and girl on top. However, there are so much more in depth positions that bring a broad range of pleasure to you and your partner. These positions are ideal for those who want to kick things up a notch in the bedroom.

☐ Yawning Position: This one is rather easy to do, but does not allow for deep penetration. It is great for a woman that is pregnant, or for the beginning of sex as you work into more complex and deep penetration positions. To do this position, have the woman lying on her back, and the male kneel between her legs. The woman should raise her legs in a V shape on either side of the man, and rest her calves on each of his sides. The eroticism of this position will make it a great turn on for both partners.

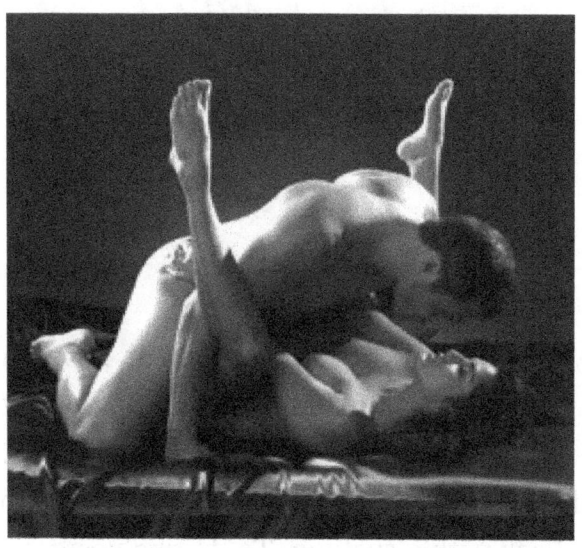

☐   Variant of the Yawning: This position should only be attempted when a woman is fully aroused due to the depth of penetration. It is easy to slip into from the yawning position, but due to the changed leg angle, allows for some really deep penetration. To do this pose, simply start in the yawning position and then have the woman move her legs up to the man's shoulders as he leans over her as if moving into the missionary position. Thrusting in this pose should not be too violent, to avoid damage to the woman's cervix.

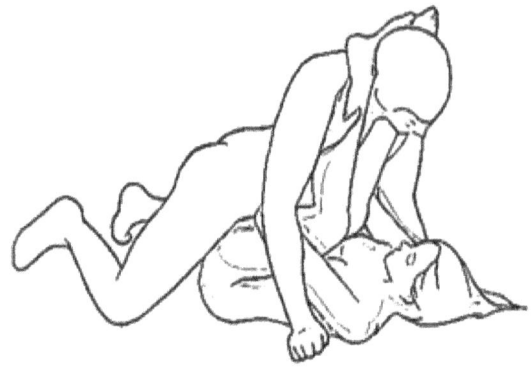

☐ Widely Open Position: This is a great position for female pleasure, as the clitoris is exposed to the friction of sex. Some females may find that keeping their back arched while being thrust against is difficult, so if you have a hard time with that, you can support your back with a cushion. To do this position, the woman lies on her back and arches up to meet her partner, with her legs spread far apart.

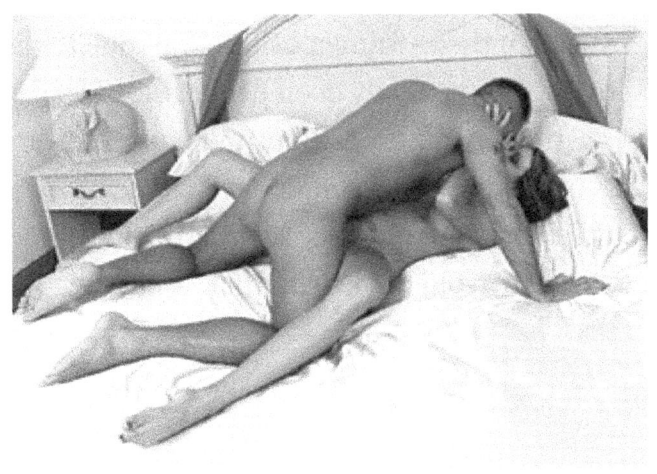

☐ The Mare's Position: This is a girl on top position that is fairly easy to do, but does require some control of the vaginal muscles to do successfully. In this position, the man sits on the edge of the bed or a chair, while the woman straddles him facing away from him with her knees bend on the surface behind her. Using her vaginal muscles and a small bouncing movement, the woman squeezes and releases the male's penis with her vagina.

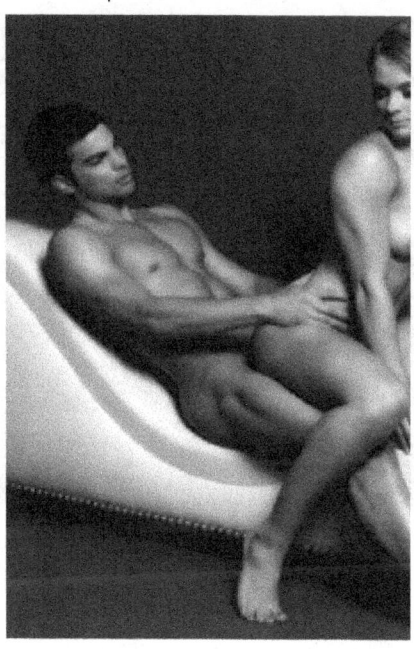

☐ Pressed Position: This is a position that is really good for a male who does not boast a significant amount of length in his penis. However, the woman must be fairly flexible for this. She must bend her knees to her chest while putting her feet against her lover's chest. He is to enter her slowly and find a speed and depth that is comfortable for both of them, due to the shortening of the vagina in this position.

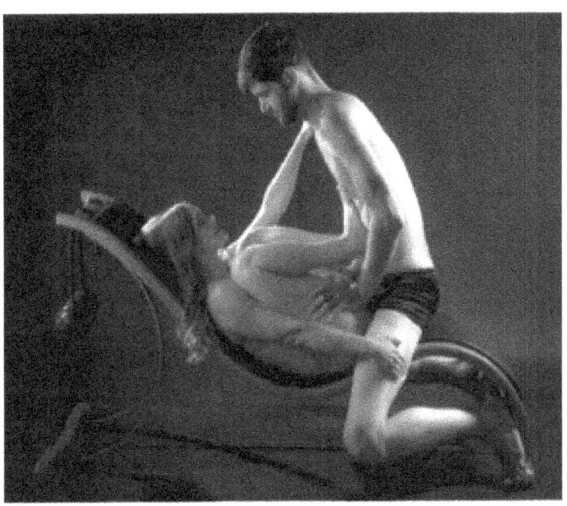

Those are five really good positions to try that does not require years of athletic training to produce. There are many other, more intense positions that require ore strength and athleticism to do, and sex should be about pleasure, not strength. Now coupled with the benefits of a more active sex life, there are a lot of benefits to the Kama sutra lifestyle that most people don't know about.

☐ Longer Life: This can actually help you live a longer life. Maybe not by twenty years, but can give you a year or two on your life span. The reason is, the more you get into it, the more sex you will have, and sex is exercise. Exercise will help extend your lifespan.

☐ Improved Mood: Along with the increases sex life, you will find that you are in a much better mood. This actually has nothing to do with the sex. It has to do with the emotional connection you will gain with your partner as you two become closer and touch and kiss more.

☐ Restful sleep: This can also help extend your life more. You will sleep better at night due to being fully worn out and satisfied, along with feeling loved and secure in your relationship as you lay next to your partner at night.

These benefits are among the many other perks of enjoying the Kama sutra life. You can use these tips whenever you like. Every night does not have to be an intense sexual encounter, but maybe on a day where you both have off, you will find that you have multiple sexual encounters. The pleasure you will find is definitely worth a little more complicated positions and learning a few new things.

Remember, you and your partner have to be comfortable with everything. You may be on board with something, but your partner may not be. You have to communicate.

Top 10 position for him

1. Cowgirl

Cowgirl is where the woman straddles the man while he's lying down and she's facing him. Why is it pleasurable for the man? The woman is doing all the work! Most of the physical movements are going to be made by the woman, but if you feel bad, you can always join in by grabbing her hips and thrusting up. This position also allows for the most penetration for a man, so it's the best stimulation for him.

If the woman is self-conscious about her body and you cannot convince her to try this position, try reverse cowgirl. It has all the same benefits for both partners, and the woman gets to show off her sexy back.

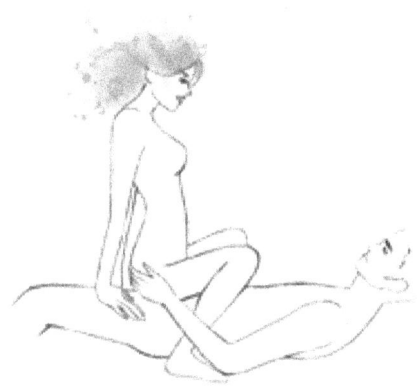

2. Around the Bend

Men love to experience deep thrusting as this is the most primal urge they have. Unfortunately, most traditional positions prevent men from going all the way in, which can leave a little something to be desired when it comes to sex for men. This position, however, alleviates all those concerns! Just position your female partner over a piece of furniture and have her spread her legs a little. Then thrust into her gently at first, and slowly build up to going into the hilt.

If the woman feels that there isn't enough intimacy, slowly lower yourself over her so that your front is touching her back. Reach around and hold her around the middle as you thrust into her to keep her steady.

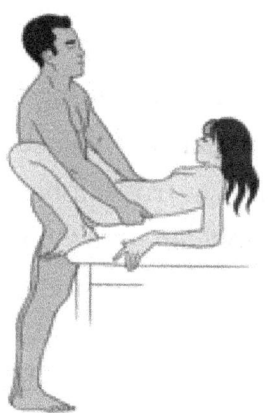

3. Inverted Rear

The man should lie down on his back and have his partner lie on top of him while she is facing the ceiling. He can grab onto her thighs and spread her legs until she's in a reverse straddle. In her position, she will not be able to do much when it comes to thrusting or moving, so the man has to do all the work. Once she's in the right position, the man can thrust as deeply as he wants, for as long as he wants.

One problem with this position is that if the sex is wild, it's difficult for the woman to stay balanced. The man can keep a firm grip on her thighs as he's thrusting to ensure she doesn't fall off.

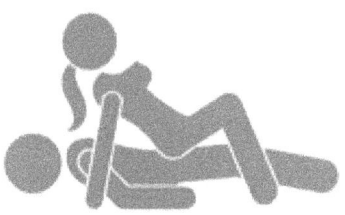

4. Full Mast

For this position, the woman is going to need to be limber. While your partner is lying on her back, place her legs at a ninety-degree angle to her body. Kneel in front of her and place her legs on your chest. Then thrust deeply and slowly until the woman is ready for more.

Sometimes, when men get a little overzealous about this position, they tend to raise the woman's back off the mattress at an odd angle. So be sure to give her extra support if this happens.

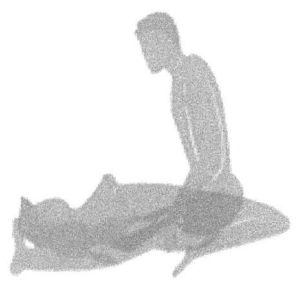

5. Lotus

Just like with the cowgirl position, this position has the woman doing almost all the work. The man sits cross-legged on the bed or on the floor and pulls her into his lap. The idea is to have the woman straddle the man with her legs around his waist, and then position herself up and down until both partners have achieved orgasm. If the woman is having trouble moving up and down, a rocking motion is just as efficient.

As a tip, have the man lean against a wall during this position. This supports his back and gives her something to hold onto, which makes it easier for her to move about.

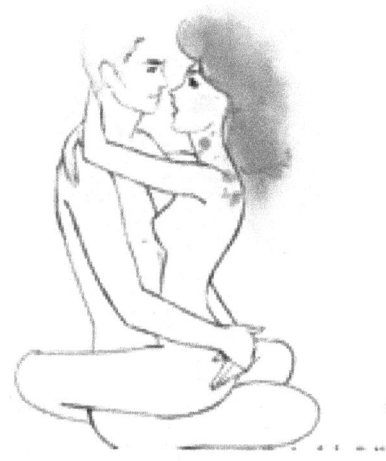

6. Doggie-Style

Doggie style is definitely the staple of a man's repertoire for dirty, naughty sex. Men get a really great view of the woman from behind and they have control over how deep and how fast they thrust during this position. It's the straight to orgasm move for a man.

Women tend to complain that they feel they're just an object during this position, and there is a lack of intimacy. That's because men tend to go through the motions and don't really get into any other kind of contact. So, men reach forward and give a gentle tug on your lady's hair or try some mild spanking.

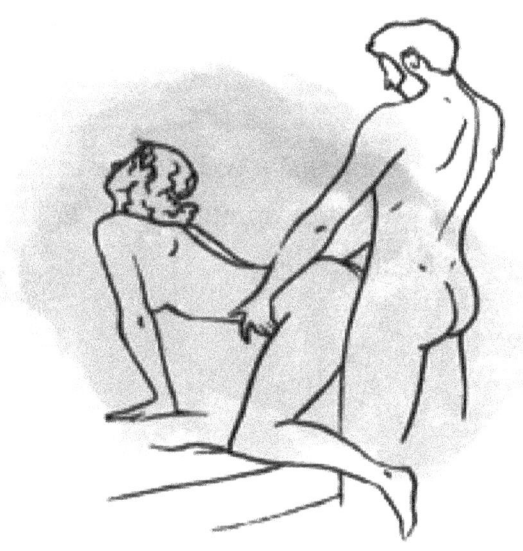

7. His Pleasure Matters!

Gentleman and ladies, a man's pleasure matters just as much as a woman's. Yes, there are positions that are more pleasurable for a woman that are not as great for a man, even if he achieves orgasm in the end. The act is not completely about the end result, but also about feeling connected and having a great time as you're getting to that orgasm. So women should be just as conscious of their man's pleasure as their man is of theirs.

Men should not be afraid to ask their partner to try something new or to focus a little on themselves at times. After all, just like women, men are responsible for their orgasms, too.

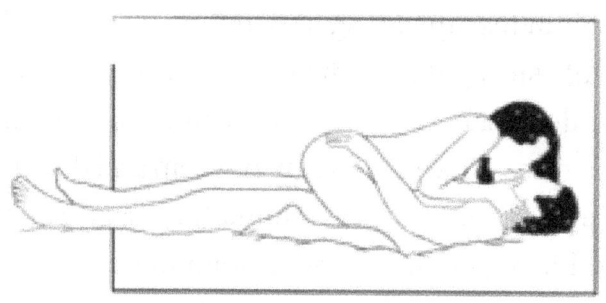

8. Packed position

The packed position is when the female extends her thighs and rests them each one on top of the other. The male can take her thighs in his arms and enter her while on his knees, kneeling.

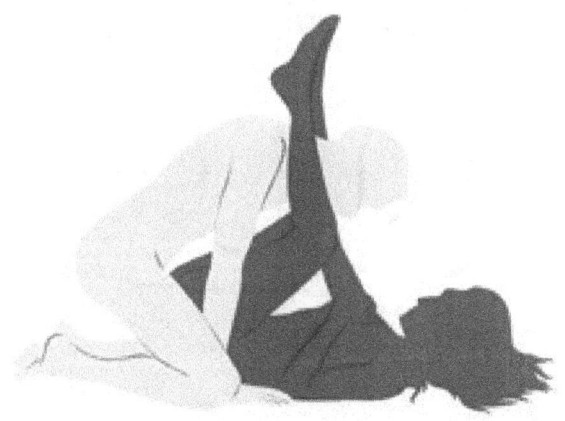

9. Lotus-like position

The lotus-like position is a highly sensual position, allowing both partners to be face to face with one another, embracing and kissing one another. The male will sit down, crossing his legs widely. The woman will sit in his lap, facing him and wrapping her legs around his back. While sitting down, she will lower herself onto his penis. This is also a deep penetration position and can be painful for men with larger penises. The woman can move up and down or back and forth while also getting clitoral stimulation from rubbing against the male's pubic region due to the positioning.

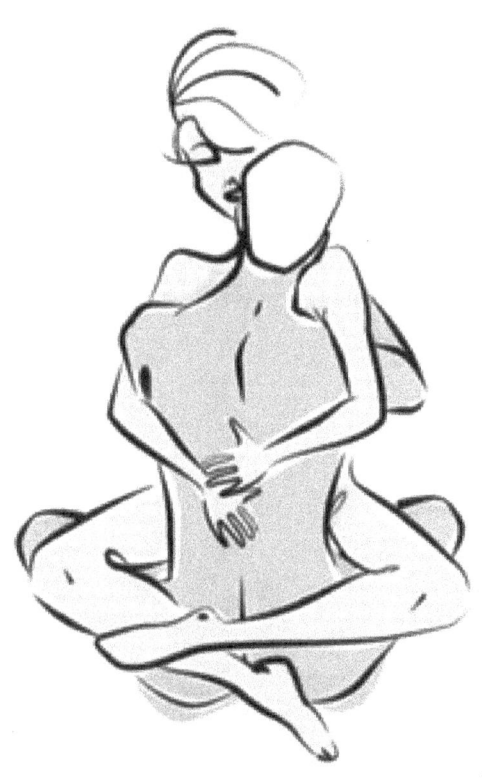

10. Turning position

Requiring a relative amount of physical strength from the male, this position has been referred to in modern times, quite accurately I might add, as "the helicopter". The man will insert himself inside the woman as if performing missionary position. From there, he will remain inside the woman while turning in a circle. Think of the woman as the body of the helicopter and the male as the top propeller for the helicopter. The penis is what is keeping this helicopter connected. This position appears to be intended more for show and experimentation than actual sexual pleasure.

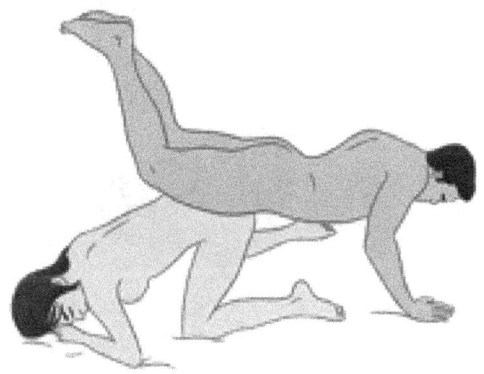

Top 10 position for her

1. Reverse Chair Sex

Think Chair Sex but with the girl facing backward, her hands holding onto the back of the chair as the male enters from behind. It has all the benefits of deep penetration but with the added excitement of falling off the chair. From this position, the guy can play with the girl's clitoris as the female holds tights to the chair. However, there may be no option to play with female hot spots since the male needs to help maintain the balance with each thrust. Most of the movement must be centered along the pelvis since a full-body thrust may topple the girl over.

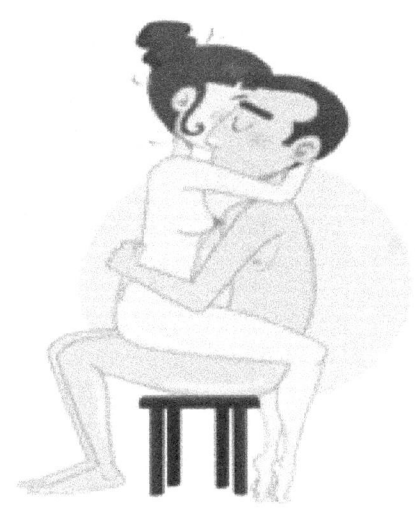

2. Climbing the Tree

Requiring balance from both the male and the female, Climbing the Tree is basically standing sex without the benefit of a wall. According to the Kama Sutra, this position provides a different kind of orgasm due to the sexual pleasure along the spine. In this situation, the male is the Tree that the female climbs with the penis acting as a branch that prevents her from falling. One of the girl's legs is hitched around the hips of the male while the other maintains balance. In this position, the male is free to play with the K-Spot, stimulate the breasts with his mouth or engage in all manners of kissing and licking.

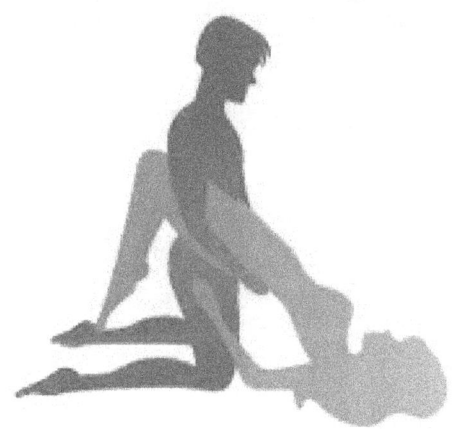

3. Almost 69

This position starts off like the Reverse Cowgirl but instead of the female staying upright, she continues to lie down to her stomach so that her face faces the feet of the male. In this position, both the girl and the boy control the movement as the female hooks her arms around the male's calves for leverage. The guy can hold onto the girl's hips to enforce more control and guide the rhythm and depth. For guys who love female ass, this is an ideal position – not to mention the fact that it lets them see the in and out movement of the penis. The only spot the guy can hit during the Almost 69 is the K-Spot although the girl can make an effort to brush her clitoris against the male with the movement.

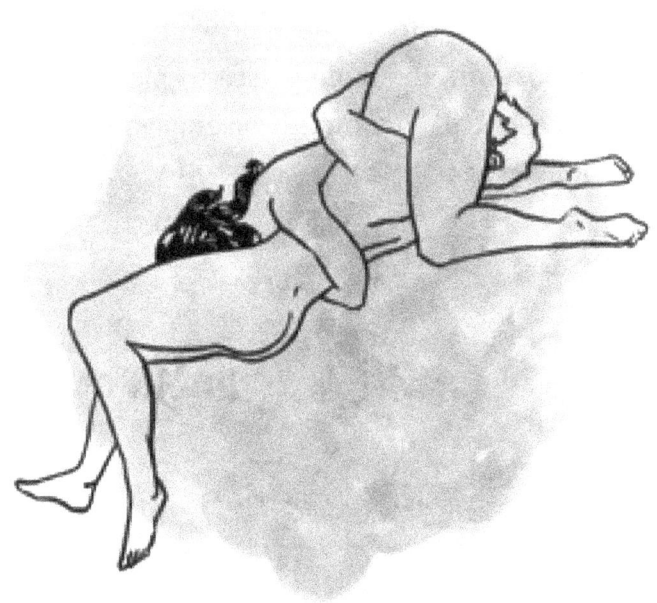

4. The Bend

Not exactly a difficult sex position, The Bend at least requires the female to be a little bit flexible. The male will also need to exert a bit more power as he bends the female's legs backward as he enters her from the front as you can see from the picture. This offers deep penetration and really keeps the vagina tight around the penis. Unfortunately, it's a little tough to hit the clitoris in this position but the female can play with her nipples in this position.

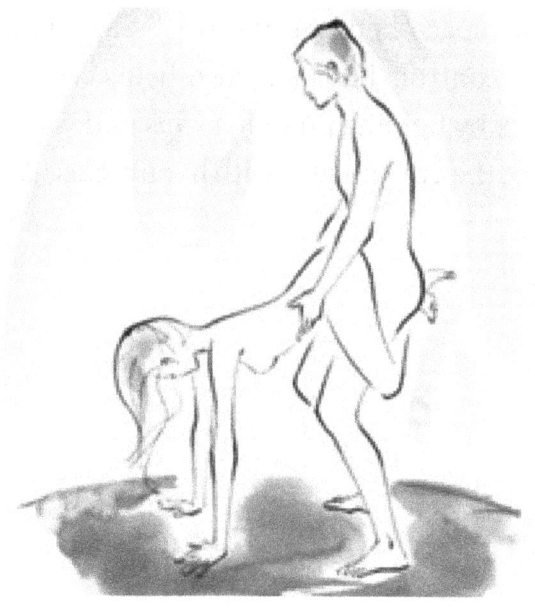

5. So Close

Have the male sit down on the bed, his thighs opened wide as the female straddles him, making them face to face. The girl then lies down on the space between the thighs and bends her knees for leverage and control. The male also helps with the depth and rhythm of the sex by holding on to her hips and waist. With a little bending forward, the guy can play with her nipples using his mouth.

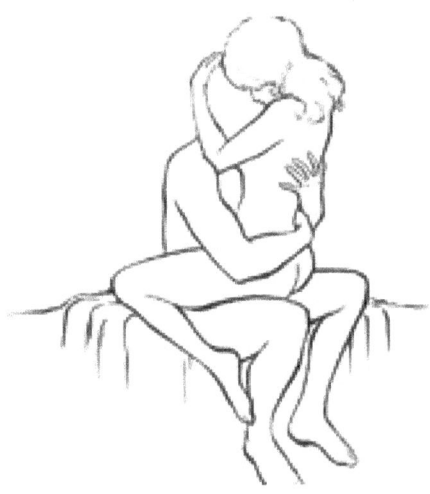

6. The Lotus

Most sexual positions require the female to be flexible but in the lotus, the male must be able to open his legs wide in a lotus position. If you've seen the position of the legs during yoga, this is exactly how it looks. The female then straddles the male, her breasts meeting his chest and getting as close as possible to effect penetration. The female wraps her thighs around the male as he controls the movement of the thrust. Women can also choose to brace their feet on the floor to help with the movement. In this position, guys can easily suck on the breasts, play with the K-Spot or perhaps do lots of smooching as they try to capture a steady rhythm to capture an orgasm. It can be tough for the guy but the open leg approach offers a different kind of pleasure for the lady. In this position, the head of the penis also gets lots of attention.

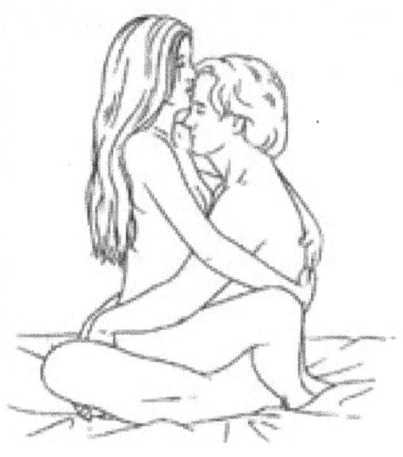

7. Pray It Out

The male kneels on the bed as the female straddles him and assumes the same kneeling position. Both are capable of controlling the thrusts but most of the works is done by the guy. In this position, couples can have one powerful kiss as the guy uses one hand to handle the K-Spot. The breasts are crushed on the guy's chest or if he's a breast man, he can also choose to suck on them as he penetrates her back and forth.

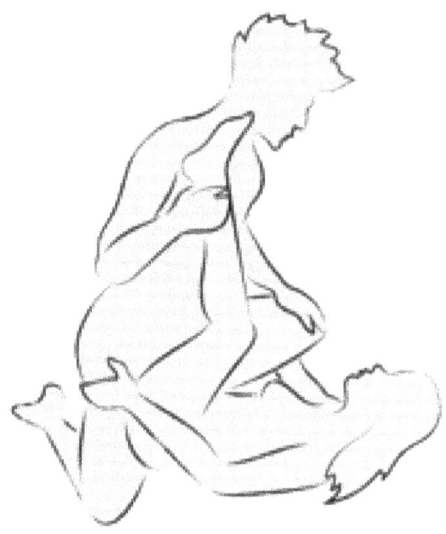

8. Doggy on Pillow

Think doggy position but more comfortable for the female as she gets down on her knees while the male enters from behind. The difference here is that the female lays down her upper body on a bunch of pillows so that she doesn't have to use her hands for leverage. In this position, the male can play with her nape, stimulating this erogenous zone until both reach orgasm. It takes a little bit of balance and control on the part of both male and female to get this position right. Also, it's not the kind of position that allows you to smack your partner with powerful thrusts so guys will need to be a little gentler in this position.

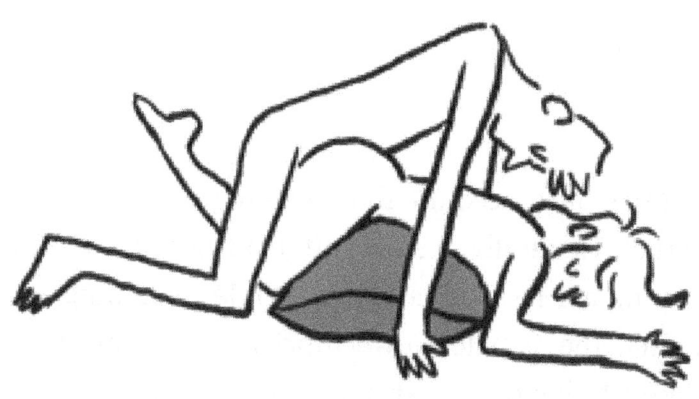

9. Flipped Almost

Think Flipped 69 but this time, with the guy taking the top space and the female occupying the bottom position. The guy does most of the work but unfortunately, this doesn't leave much room for additional stimulation. Girls, however, can massage the buttocks of their partner and if they happen to be sensitive in this area, then it will definitely be a plus. If you can, try playing with the balls as they become exposed in this position. A lot of girls, however, aren't exactly fond of the view this position provides.

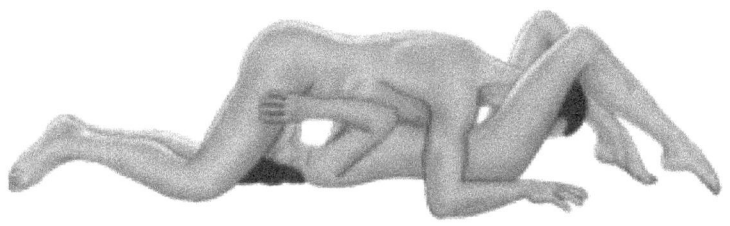

10.   Pivot

The pivot takes into account the changing of the position from one to another. Generally, it starts off in a Doggy Position with the female keeping her legs spread open. While remaining embedded in the vagina, the female slowly uprights her upper body and the male adjusts his own posture, slowly bending backward and bracing his hands on the bed to accommodate their combined weight. In this position, the knees remain bent and as much as possible; the penis remains lodged in the vagina. The female's feet are now firmly planted on the bed, her hands stretched backward and holding onto the male arms for balance as they continue their sexual thrusting. In this position, the female is free to play with her breasts or clitoris. If capable, the guy can try bracing with just one hand and use the other for pleasure giving to his partner.

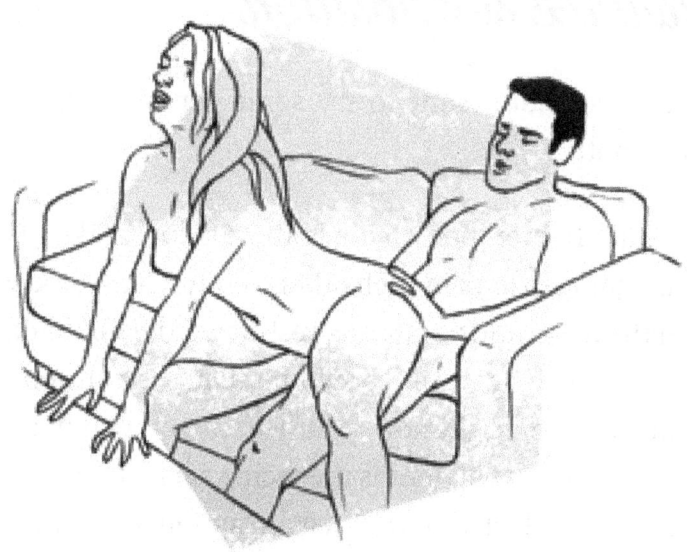

Advance sex position

Advance sex position: want to try some senior class sex styles? Check these out:

☐   Crab walk: Remember what a crab walk looks like? That's just how you are going to look in each other's body. Get seated with your feet flat on the floor, and your arms resting on the floor behind your back. Did that? Your partner should be seated right opposite you, in the same posture. Right now, your legs are arched in a 45degree position, and your sexual organs are facing each other. Move closer to each other and intertwine your legs. Your left leg on his right and his right leg on your left hip. Help his penis to find his way, it is a ravishing position!

☐   Passion propeller: this is a really advance sex game. Lie flat on your back as your man lies straight on you. guess what? The other way! He lies on you with his head towards your feet and his butt towards your breasts. His legs would be spread apart beside your pelvis and he would bend on. Imagine that sort of penetration!

☐   The X-rated: how about the other version of 'passion propeller'? absolutely possible! here is your guy flat on the floor; face up for sure. You lie flat on him, and your legs spread beside his body, while your pelvis and breast rest on his legs. Guide the daddy into the hole, do the rocking!

Powerful sex position for male orgasm & for female orgasm

The following are sex positions you could try to help your partner max out their orgasm:

1.   Powerful Sex Position for male orgasm: Try the following positions to help your male partner reach a faster orgasm;

☐   Blowjob: You do blowjobs by putting your partner's penis straight in your mouth. Drive it in and out with a controlled precision. Massage it gently with your lips and watch pure delight on his face as he ejaculates.

☐   Doggy style: You surely remember the get-on all four sex style. It allows a man to maximize his thrust which can in turn, lead to a commanding orgasm.

☐   Barrow style: Do you remember the seated barrow style? Try it more often and compare it with any other style your partner enjoys. You shouldn't be surprised that your partner loves the barrow style than the others.

2.   Powerful sex position for female orgasm:

☐ Scissoring: Can you imagine forming a scissor with your lover? It is pretty simple, and it is one of the most guaranteed to make her multiple orgasm if done correctly. She only needs to lay on one side while one of her legs is raised towards your shoulder. You are kneeling between her legs. You can suck that toe and send a shiver of sensation into her. The toe is an erogenous spot. You are at that same time penetrating the vagina. Remembering your two hands are free? The clit, the nipples, they are up for your stimulation. You are exploring more than two of her sensual spots. Her orgasm will be a blast!

☐   Doggy style: Amazing! Doggy style again. Remember you are penetrating her from the rear and your hands are completely free. You can give an erotic massage to the nipples with a free hand and her clit with the other. Pretty hard? Just the first time. It brings you closer to each other as you would likely lie on her back while trying to achieve this stimulation. Imagine how close you would be! Her orgasm would be superb too.

Role play

Role Play is a fun and exciting way to step outside of yourselves and try something new in your sex life. If you have been together for a while and are very comfortable with each other and in your sexual routines, role-playing is a way to try something new. Role-playing allows you to be different people while still having sex with each other exclusively. It is a fun way to act out your wildest fantasies and can help you both to try things you might be shy or nervous to do normally. Hiding behind the role you are playing may give you that confidence boost you need.

Role-play can look different to every couple, it all depends on what you like and what you want to try. You can get creative with the relationships between your characters and have fun with it. We are going to look at some examples of role plays you can try if you are new to the idea and want to know where and how to get started.

Keep in mind that classic rules of what is okay and what is not in terms of the relationships between the characters do not apply in role-play situations. The rule that a teacher and student cannot have sex doesn't matter when you and your partner are alone and are turning each other on. It is all about fantasy, so try to let yourself settle into this idea and it will allow you to get into it and really let yourself be turned on by whatever you find turns you on, even if it wouldn't exist in the real world, outside of your bedroom.

Sex game

Having fun and playing dirty can bring an unimaginable color to your sexual life. Have you ever wondered how glamorous your sex would look if you add more fun to it? Imagine you and your partner having a very hot intercourse, laughing and playing hard before and after. Do you think anyone would even a pain that may have generated from the sex? If you ask me, the difference between consensual sex and rape is fun.

Sex itself is fun, but it could be more fun when you add a bit to it. it can also stick you with your partner forever. They would imagine how it was always fun with you, how it would be very hard to get someone else to understand them or start the fun with them. Naturally, using a sexual style like this is excellent for a partner you are trying to win their heart.

Oral sex

Phew! Let's talk about the 21st century sex! Oral sex is among the most popular sex types that grow in 21st century. It's not a new invention, that is certain, but it is hardly considered a proper sex style until 21st century.

Till date, some cultures and communities still think it is a bad idea to give oral sex to a sexual partner, even your wife. This is a completely personal decision, and nobody can blame you for it. Some folks have gone beyond these personal sentiments however. They are excited by the prospect of licking their partner or having their partner link them deep down. So, they really want to try it, but they need some ideas and they want to be sure this is safe. Does that sound like you? Awesome, let's talk about some interesting facts about oral sex.

What is oral sex itself? The sexual act of having your partner's genitals in your mouth, on your tongue or in between your lips rather than putting their genital in your mouth or gunning to fill their hole all the time. Now, you understand that you may perform oral sex on your male or female partner.

From all angles you may choose to analyze it, oral sex has been endorsed by standard medical researches across the world. It has been analyzed as 'safe' for anyone to try when they feel the desire to. There are always precautions to take as you would expect, there are also important lessons to learn in each instance.

Sexual variant

Major sexual variations

Exhibitionism is among the most common of the sexual variations. The usual image is of a middle aged man in a dirty raincoat "flashing." Typically, however, exhibitionists are post pubescent males up to the age of 40 who obtain high levels of sexual pleasure and excitement from exposing their genitals to females, usually strangers, and who may masturbate at the same time.

Paedophilia involves intense sexual urges and sexual activity with prepubescent children. Two thirds of molested children are girls, usually between the ages of 8 and 11. To meet the diagnostic criteria, a paedophile must be at least 16 years old and at least five years older than the victim. Most paedophiles are men, but there are cases of women having repeated sexual contact with children. In 90% of cases the molester is known to the child, and 15% (possibly more) are relatives. Most paedophiles are heterosexual and are often married with their own children, although they commonly have marital or sexual difficulties or problems with alcohol misuse. Eighty per cent have a history of childhood sexual abuse.

Fetishism involves recurrent sexual urges or behaviors concerning the use of inanimate objects such as leather and rubber garments, women's underwear, stockings, and shoes and boots.

Transvestism refers to recurrent, intense sexually arousing fantasies, urges, and behaviors involving cross dressing. A transvestite is a heterosexual male who derives sexual satisfaction by wearing female clothing. Many are married and seem very masculine. They should not be mistaken for female impersonators on the stage (such as "Dame Edna Everage") or male homosexuals who cross dress ("go in drag"), who are not sexually aroused or dependent on their cross dressing for sexual excitement.

Transsexualism is not, strictly speaking, a paraphilia but rather an issue of gender role. Transsexuals have an intense desire to become a member of the opposite sex, feeling that they are trapped in the "wrong body." Many therefore ask for surgical intervention for a sex change. Transsexualism is found equally in males and females, and they should not be confused with transvestites, who cross dress for sexual arousal but who do not want anatomical change.

Hypoxyphilia is an increasingly commonly reported variation that involves attempts to enhance the pleasure of orgasm by a reduction of oxygen intake—for example, by placing a tight noose around one's neck. Such behavior has led to fatalities.

Other sexual variations include gaining sexual pleasure from inflicting pain (sadism) or from suffering pain or humiliation (masochism), sexual desire for corpses (necrophilia) or for animals (zoophilia or bestiality), arousal from contact with urine (urophilia) and faeces (coprophilia), and excitement from rubbing the genitals against a clothed person in a confined space such as the Underground (frotteurism).

Combinations—It is not unusual for an individual to have more than one sexual variation. The commonest combination is fetishism, transvestism, sadism, and masochism.

Sexual variations seen in clinical settings are only a proportion of the cases where such problems exist. There are, broadly speaking, four classes of clinical referral.

• Those sent for clinical intervention by the law enforcing authorities. These are sex offenders who are asked to have treatment to help them overcome their problem behavior.

Those who seek help for their sexual variations because they are distressed by them. These include people who worry that they might commit illegal or embarrassing acts. Many are distressed by acts they see as "unnatural" or are afraid that they may endanger their life or their career.

Those who seek help because their partners are distressed by the sexual variation. They are themselves distressed because of their partner's distress. These are people with stable or long term relationships.

Those who present with frank sexual dysfunction. They report erectile difficulties or other dysfunctions, which are usually secondary to strong variant desires and reliance on these for arousal. For example, a man may find that he is unable to sustain an erection for sexual intercourse with his partner unless he has contact with, say, a leather garment.

Anal sex

Anal sex isn't something that everyone wishes to try, but if you are someone who is open to seeing what it's all about and why people like it. Anal sex can be enjoyed by everyone, any combination of genders and genitals. Anal sex is commonly associated with gay men and straight men may be intimidated by the thought of being penetrated, but many men in heterosexual relationships enjoy being pegged by their female partners with a dildo or strap-on. This can be for couples with vaginas using a strap-on, couples with penises or couples with a combination of both. Pleasure is universal and so are these positions!

There are a few things to go keep in mind before beginning. The key to anal sex is lubrication! You will need to make sure that both the penis (or dildo) and the anus are well-lubricated in order for anal sex to be pleasurable for everyone involved. The anus doesn't lubricate itself like the vagina does, so you have to make sure you do it yourselves before sex. The next point to keep in mind is relaxation. The anus will open gradually as you start to play around and inside it a little bit, and as you slide something into it, so having the person be relaxed and comfortable is very important. Remember to let it do its thing, and just slowly enjoy the process without rushing it. The next thing to note is that if you are going to remove something like a toy or a penis from the anus, it is important to make sure the person is relaxed, lubricated and expecting it to happen. If you try to quickly remove it without the person expecting it, their body will reflexively tense the anus and it will lead to a painful experience, possibly for both of you. Remembering these three points will help you to have a positive and enjoyable anal sex experience.

How to Use Hands

Now that you have learned a variety of new Kama Sutra positions ranging from semi-advanced to extreme-level advanced, we are going to switch gears for a moment and look at ways that you can arouse your partner and bring them to orgasm only using your hands. This is possible for both men and women; the techniques you use just may be slightly different. This, to you, may seem reminiscent of middle school where you used only your hands and never went further than that. Remember those "did you finger her?" "did you give him a hand job?" days? This may be true. However, there is skill involved in being able to arouse and bring your partner to orgasm using only your hands.

Massage

One way to do this is by giving them a massage all over their body using some warm massage oil and work your way to their genitals. Move slowly and let the sexual frustration build inside of them.

Alternatively, you can begin immediately without a massage and by only using your hands on their genitals. There are some benefits to using only your hands as they can feel their way around, so you know exactly what you are doing and there is no guesswork involved. You can control the pressure with which you hold or stroke their penis, or rub their clitoris. You can feel your way around inside of them so you know exactly where you are and can aim for a specific type of orgasm such as prostate, G-Spot, deeper vaginal, or clitoral.

Toys and accessories

Sex with toys can bring a new element of mystery and novelty to your sex life. It comes with new sensations and added pleasures that you may not have experienced before. Knowing where to start with toys in a world with countless varieties of uses, shapes, and sizes can be overwhelming at first, but here you will get an overview of where you can start and what positions you can use them in!

Vibrator

A vibrator can make a woman orgasm very intensely and in quite a short amount of time if her partner knows how to use it for her. When figuring out what your woman likes and how she likes to use her vibrator, make her the center of attention.

The Queen

Begin with her lying down on her back on the bed, relaxed and ready to receive your gifts of pleasure. Place yourself close to her genitals in a position that is comfortable and leaves your hands and arms free to move. You can try sitting cross-legged beside her or lying perpendicular to her, halfway down her body with the vibrator in your hand and the other hand free to roam. Start off very slow and gentle and find her clitoris with your fingers. Turn the vibrator on a low buzz, slowly bring it between her legs and place it so that it lightly touches her clitoris.

Strap-On

A strap-on is another toy that can be used in a variety of ways to enhance your pleasure and your sex life. It is more common than you may imagine that in heterosexual sex, the woman will wear a strap-on and pleasure her male partner anally with it. This is called Pegging. While it is not for everyone, many men find pleasure from this because of the sensitivity of their prostate and many women find pleasure from this because they can see their man reaching higher levels of pleasure than ever before. This may be something you want to try.

Another situation where this toy would be a great inclusion would be in a lesbian relationship or two-vagina sex of any sort for that matter. One partner can wear the strap-on to penetrate the other partner either anally or vaginally.

Strap-On Doggy Style Anal Sex

Quite a mouthful to say, this position is a combination of a few other positions we have seen thus far. This position brings them all together to create a mecca of pleasure. Doggy style can be done with a strap-on to penetrate someone vaginally as we have seen already, but here we are going to look at Doggy Style Anal Sex.

Vibrating Ring

A Vibrating Cock Ring can be an amazing tool to take both male and female sex up a notch. The vibrating ring goes over the man's penis and down to the bottom of his shaft. This heightens his pleasure and he can use it during masturbation, but can also heighten the woman's pleasure when it is used during penetration. Sharing this with someone else during vaginal or anal sex can help you both have better orgasms. The other benefit of this ring is that it does not just enhance female pleasure from the vibrations it causes on the man's penis while it is inside of her, but also from the vibration it can give to the woman's clitoris when used in certain positions. The position we will examine is one that will benefit the female's clitoris.

Vibrating Ring Seated

With the Cock Ring positioned at the base of your penis and vibrating away, sit down in a chair and place your feet on the floor. It is preferable to use a chair with no armrests for more ease in this position and one that is lower to the ground. If you don't have one like this, a regular kitchen chair or a stool placed in front of a wall will work just fine. Have the woman sit on your lap facing you with her legs around your waist and behind you, touching the floor if she can for more support. Have her stand up slightly so she is hovering over you and lower her onto your rock hard, vibrating penis.

Double-Ended Dildo

A double-ended dildo may seem like an intimidating sex toy, especially if you are a male-female couple. As a man, you may never have used something like this before. As a woman, you may wonder why you would. Understanding how this toy can enhance your sex life and add many new dimensions to both of your pleasure will unlock a whole new world of sex for both of you. A double-ended dildo can be used on a variety of occasions and in a variety of positions, but the position we are going to talk about here is the classic male-female pegging, only this time with a double-ended toy.

The Double-Ended Pillar

Start with lots of lube (like any anal position) and when both people are adequately hard/wet. Have your man lie down on his stomach on a soft surface and begin by woman sitting on his butt with your legs on either side of him, facing his feet. Warm-up his butthole a little bit by using your tongue or your fingers to tease it. This will get it ready and also will tease him just enough to have him begging for more.

Chapter 10

Periods and Sex

There are some benefits that come from having sex on your period. One of these benefits is that having sex while on your period can actually offer relief from the pain of period cramps. Period cramps can be very painful, and anything that makes them feel better is a welcome suggestion, especially when it feels as good as sex will. This result is because of the orgasm. The chemicals that are released in the brain make you feel happy and also have pain relief functions. The other reason is that an orgasm makes the uterus contract and then release. The release part of this will likely make a woman feel better than she did before in terms of cramps.

Another benefit of having an orgasm during your period is that it leads to the uterus contracting, which actually pushes the blood and uterus contents out faster, leading to a shorter period length. This also means that there is ample natural lubrication and that lubricant is not necessary during period sex.

Best Kama Sutra Positions to Try During Menstruation

A good way to have sex during menstruation is in the shower. This makes it so that there is not much cleanup involved, and the blood that gets on either of you will be able to be washed off right away. This is a cleaner and more comfortable alternative to having sex in bed and having to jump in the shower afterward. Additionally, shower sex is steamy (literally) and hot (literally) and can make for some very fun body-on-body action. Make sure the water is the perfect temperature and that you have a mat or something on the floor so you aren't slipping all over the place! Before you start any type of penetration in the water, make sure you use lots of waterproof lube because the water in the shower won't be enough of a lubricant for the inside of a vagina and will actually make for some painful friction. Let's avoid that; lube is your friend!

Standing Doggy Style

Standing Doggy Style is a position from the Kama Sutra with a twist. It is a good place to start with shower sex because it will make sure that you don't get sprayed in the face with a hot stream of water while you are trying to focus on having a blissful orgasm. Pleasurable for both parties, Doggy Style in the shower is a new take on an old favorite.

The man stands with his back to the running water with the woman standing in front of him, facing away from him. The woman then bends forward and can put her hands on the edge of the tub or the wall of the shower for support. The man slides his penis into her from behind, grabbing onto her hips for a deeper thrust, and then they are ready to go for it. This position has a good chance of the man being able to hit the woman's G-spot with his penis, so this position will be greatly enjoyed by the woman. The warmth and the wet environment of the shower are sure to make for an unforgettable sexual encounter.

Kama Sutra Shower Sex Position

This is another position to try in the shower. If you both are in the mood for a position that doesn't need you to focus too much on difficult positioning and holding yourselves up in a slippery shower, you can try the kneeling position. Have yourselves kneel on the floor of the shower, one person behind the other? From here, you can go in many different ways. You can use this position as foreplay as you both reach around to pleasure the other's genitals with your hands before you move to the bedroom together. You can also use this as foreplay before switching to another position for penetration in the shower. Or you can start penetration right away. For penetration, you will have to adjust each of your heights on your knees to line up your erection and her vagina to meet nicely for smooth penetration. This position is full of possibilities and is a very hot way to get you both in the mood for whatever is to come either in the shower or out of it.

Bouncy Chair

This is not a shower position, but it is a great position for having sex during your period. This is because it can be done on the floor so that you can more easily clean up afterward.

To get into this position, the man will get on his knees on the floor (on towels or sheets for ease of cleaning) and sit back on his heels. The woman will sit on his lap, facing him, and put his penis inside of her. She will keep her feet planted on the floor and use the balls of her feet to bounce herself up and down on the man's penis. This position is great because the woman is hovering over the floor and this will allow for most of the blood to land there instead of all over the bed or the man.

Things to Keep in Mind

There are a few things to keep in mind if you and your partner decide that you wish to have sex on your period.

1.   Blood Stains

Ensure that before you begin, if you are going to have sex anywhere outside of the bathtub or the shower, that you put down a lot of towels or something that will be able to absorb the blood. If you get it on your white bed sheets, it will stain. Keep I mind as well that whatever towels you choose to lay down will also likely be stained, so be sure to choose those that you don't need to keep freshly white.

2.   Self-Consciousness

Having sex during her period may make a woman feel self-conscious. Keeping this in mind is important as she may feel sensitive about her body or the amount of blood that is involved.

3.   Sexually Transmitted Infections

One thing that is important to note is that there are some STIs that are transmitted through the blood. These are HIV or hepatitis. In order to stay safe, it is important to use condoms all the time, but especially when there will be blood involved during sex.

4.   Tampons

Tampons that are forgotten about when having sex can cause a problem. If you were wearing a tampon before having sex, ensure that you remove it before a penis or fingers are inserted into the vagina. Otherwise, the tampon will need to be removed by a doctor.

5.   You Can Still Get Pregnant

While the chances are lower during your period, you can still become impregnated during your period. It is difficult to say at what point your body will be ready to conceive during your period, so taking adequate precautions is necessary.

Chapter 11

Sex in pregnancy

Sex Positions for When You Are Pregnant

If you are pregnant, congratulations! Luckily, despite conflicting theories and rumors surrounding this topic, you are still able to have sex while you are pregnant. If you have a special case and are unsure about having sex, ask your doctor for advice. In terms of the common myths about pregnancy like "will my penis touch the baby?" or "will it rupture the placenta?" The answer to these questions is a big N-O and these fears should not prevent you from enjoying and orgasm for the entirety of your nine-month pregnancy.

The best positions for sex when you are pregnant will depend on how far along in your pregnancy you are, because the size of your belly, your flexibility, and your general mobility will change as you enter the stages of pregnancy. Very early on, in the first trimester, for example, you can do virtually any sex positions you like because your belly will still be quite small and so will the baby, which means neither will be big enough for any certain position to affect them yet. When you begin showing, and your belly is increasing in size from this point on, you will want to take some things into consideration when it comes to sex positions, mostly for your own comfort!

When you are pregnant, this could actually be the best time in your life for sex in terms of your orgasms and overall pleasure! Having sex during pregnancy will actually feel better than ever before because there will be many sex hormones coursing through your veins at all times. This means that your entire vaginal area will have even more blood flow than usual- especially when you are aroused, and your nipples will be extra sensitive. Your man will feel the positive effects of this too because your vagina will be extra lubricated and engorged. This will not only lead to more pleasure for you when he is inside of you, but it will feel amazing for him as well because of the tighter space he will be sliding his penis into. Some women even say that they are able to reach orgasm much easier, or for the first time ever when they have pregnant sex! It is said that the second trimester is the best time of the forty weeks of your pregnancy for sex in terms of pleasure. At this stage your morning sickness is no longer rampant, your body is feeling the positive effects of all of those hormones floating around, and your belly isn't too big to restrict your movement or your flexibility too much just yet.

It is said that you should not lie on your back after the 20th week of pregnancy and all of the sex positions that follow will accommodate that. Lying on your back during pregnancy can close off access to an important nerve for you and the baby, but fear not- you will feel the discomfort if this is happening and you can adjust accordingly.

In general, the best positions will be those that avoid putting pressure on your belly-which would be uncomfortable for you and your partner likely, and positions that will keep you off of your back. The most comfortable ones for you will avoid both of these things anyway, so make sure your comfort is the first priority when it comes to sex during pregnancy.

Hot Seat

The first position we will talk about is the Hot Seat. This position is good for the first or second trimester when you are still very mobile and only starting to show a little bit of a baby bump.

The man sits upright on the edge of the bed with his legs hanging off and his feet on the floor. Sit down onto his lap, facing away from him and slide his penis into you. You can shift your body around and see which angle feels the best for both of you. Your man can reach around you and massage your nipples or play with your clit from this position as well, and he can kiss your neck and back sensually. You can move as slow or as fast as you like in this position, and take it at the depth you like. This is good for those days when your morning sickness just won't give up.

Spooning

Spooning is a great position for sex when you are pregnant because it allows you and your partner to get super close without having a large belly in between you, and it has you in an optimal position for comfort. As your pregnancy progresses, you may become more swollen and less mobile in general, so having your partner do most of the work during sex is ideal.

Begin by lying on your side in a comfortable position. Your partner is lying on their side as well, and he comes up behind you pressing his body against yours. From here, he can slide into you from behind and reach around you to gently massage your body or whisper sweet nothings into your ear. He does the thrusting into you with his hips and can hold onto yours for support.

This position allows you to feel relaxed and supported and doesn't require much of anything to get into. This position is great for some weekend morning sex or sex after a long day when you horny but too tired to maneuver your bigger body.

Sideways

This position is good for all of the reasons that I mentioned above (Lying on your side, your partner doing the work) as well as giving you the opportunity to see each other's faces. Your partner may also be able to get deeper in this position because he can slide his body down towards your legs and get his hips further in between yours this way. To make it easier, you can bend the knee of your upper leg and point it towards the ceiling as much as you are able to. Your partner will be able to slide his hips in here between your legs with ease and reach a deeper penetration if that is what you're after.

Tabletop

Sit on a table or counter and lean back so that your weight is supported on your arms behind you. Spread your legs wide. Have your partner stand in front of the table between your legs and slide his penis into you from the front. You can lean back and relax while your partner does the thrusting with his hips.

This position is good for pregnancy sex because you can adjust the angle of your upper body according to the size of your belly and lean in a position that is comfortable for you. You get to recline while being penetrated without fully lying on your back and you are supported by the table instead of trying to hold a position on a squishy bed. Give this one a try and play around with angles. If it is uncomfortable for you for whatever reason, try this on the edge of your bed instead with your partner standing in front of it. If you cannot hold yourself up with your arms behind you, prop a bunch of pillows behind you to hold your body up at a similar angle.

Cowgirl

The classic Cowgirl position looks like the following: The man lies on his back on the bed and you climb on top of him, straddling him at the waist and facing his upper body. You sit on his penis, sliding it into you.

Once in this position, continue riding his erection at your pace. You can control the depth, the speed, and the angle. Find what's most comfortable for you and adjust it as you go through your pregnancy and your body changes. Your man gets to enjoy looking at your beautiful belly and can even play with your clitoris here.

The key to pregnant sex is comfort ability. Listen to your body and be aware of what feels different as you progress through it. If something doesn't feel great, try another position. Everyone's pregnancy is different and everyone will have a different level of flexibility and range of motion. What is comfortable for one couple may not work for another and vice-versa. Be sure to enjoy the benefits of all of those sex hormones though, it will be as if you are a horny teenager all over again but with the benefits of adulthood!

Take full advantage of the time that you have pre-baby as well because it will prove to be more difficult to find the time and space to have sex once you have a child. It is not necessary to give up on sex when you add a baby into your life, but you have to be strategic with your sex life.

Chapter 12

Sex in overweight

There are various ways that you could make your sex life enjoyable if you or your partner is overweight. Nothing should stop you from getting the best out of your partner through positivity and exploration. The first step about enjoying intimacy in your relationship should be disregarding the misconception associated with being overweight. Notably, issues arise in case one or all partners are overweight. You should find the best way to overcome those acts not only as a motivation but also a strong bond in the relationship. The following are considerations that you should make if you want to enjoy sex with an overweight partner.

1.   Be positive: With the acceptance that there is little you could do to change the situation, you are sure to find better ways to make your sex life more intimate. In addition, there should be no misconceptions to hinder you from making love to your partner as long as you are sure that they would enjoy it. Living positively

and developing attitudes to support your life will make you most romantic to your partner.

2.   Own your Body Size: You should not live in denial over the size of your body, thinking that it would prove unromantic to your partner. Note that being overweight does not make you ugly but makes you beautiful, depending on your partner's perception. For that reason, you should accept that you are overweight and be proud of it in order to make others find the beauty in you. Similarly, you should make your partner feel the same as they are overweight to alter their perception and eventually improve self-esteem.

3.   Take Time: The fact that your partner is overweight does not mean that they are different in their sex life. You should serve them in the same manner as you would treat a slim partner. In this case, you should take time when having sex with your partner, involving all the steps that are usually engaged in sex. Do not focus only on penetration, but you should take time for foreplay, and other forms of stimulation ton turn them on.

4.   Handle with Pride: It is common to find sagging and loose body part in overweight people, making you confused about how to react. It should not turn you off as it is the sole reason they f classified as overweight. You should treat the body parts as sensitive and needing a stimulating touch for sexual arousal. These parts include the buttocks, thighs, and the pubis. They are the most sensitive parts in obese people and may be the source of sexual stimulation and orgasm if caressed or rubbed.

5.   No Desperation: As an overweight partner, you should not show desperation due to your body size for it may hinder you from achieving sexual satisfaction. Instead, you should be content with

yourself and make the best out of the activity. Expect to be treated as any other partner and believe that you deserve the best for you do. Therefore, live within your means and find happiness and pleasure whenever your partner means to introduce them to you.

6.   Position: There positions that might be difficult to try out for overweight couples. However, you could also explore additional positions that would help you attain orgasm and experience great intimacy. For example, the reverse cowgirl is perfect for it puts the bellies at different positions, making it easy6 for the woman on top to control the movement and penetration.

7.   Additional Requirements: Overweight people require platforms that would support their total weight, especially when making angles and moves involved in intimacy. For that reason, you should outsource better equipment to enhance your sex life and feel relaxed whenever you jump into action. You require pillows to position your partner to make little efforts in the attempt of making sexual advances and stimulation. Similarly, you may need spring surfaced to balance your weights and reduce bodily friction.

8.   Maintain Intimacy: There is no reason to leave your partner due to overweight or obesity. Various factors may have contributed to the condition, and it would be for your own good. Therefore, it is advisable to keep the love and intensify intimacy to make them feel appreciated and cherished. With the realization that sex is enjoyable in overweight, you would need to keep on having sex with your partner.

Pros of Sex in Overweight

•   Exercise: Sexual activity is part of an exercise, for it involves body movements and application of pressure. Overweight partners can regulate their body mass index when they engage in sex, thus improving body performance.

• Boosts Moods: Overweight people have difficulties managing their moods primarily due to the isolation and stigmatization they may face from society. Therefore they require attention and cuddling to rejuvenate the affection. Sex offers these advantages and helps them rethink their negativity.

• Aids the Immune System: Sexual engagement among the overweight plays a significant role in enhancing their immune system. Orgasm helps release hormones used by the immune system to fight conditions in the body.

• Regulates Blood Pressure: Sexual activities and orgasm involve a robust circulation of blood throughout the body. As a result, the body maintains a healthy blood pressure preventing you from blood pressure-related conditions.

• Boosts Self-Esteem: The act of caressing, cuddling, and penetrating an overweight partner may prove to be a great feeling for them, especially if they had faced isolation or stigmatization. They feel adored and find their value when they satisfy their partners sexually.

• Long-Lasting: Being overweight is known to cause long term reaction among men. It might result in total satisfaction of the partner contrary to other men who last for seconds, leaving their partners hanging in sexual desperation.

• Bonding: Intimate relationship among the overweight

enhances the mutual bond and creates a loving environment for the partners. As a result, the partners remain connected, promising an enjoyable sex life ahead.

Cons

• Positioning: Overweight partners may experience difficulties trying out various positions that may help them attain the utmost intimacy. The limited flexibility hinders the performance of positions such as 69. However, there are positions to try out as you advance to more complex ones.

• Low Performance: Being overweight may hinder stamina development. It makes it impossible for partners to acquire physical strength that is vital in maintaining positions and keeping the orgasm longer. As a result, the partner may feel dissatisfied in sexual intercourse, leaving them in desperation.

Best Positions for Sex in Overweight

• Reverse Cowgirl: In this position, the man lies flat on a bed as the woman turns while facing the same direction as the man. It helps the man make great stimulation on the G-spot while minimizing the contact between the bellies. Similarly, it allows the woman to take full control of the depth and pace of penetration.

• Doggy: It is also a reverse version where the man penetrates from behind. The woman may bend and lean on a walk or any other platform for support. The position exposes the anus and the vagina to the man making it easy for him to access the clitoris and holding on her.

• Missionary: The numerous variants of this position makes it easy to have sex with an overweight partner. The woman may lift her legs to place them on the shoulders of the man correctly placing the clitoris for stimulation from the pelvis of the man. You could also p by placing the woman on the edge of a bed as the man stands supporting her legs and making thrusts.

• Anal: It is a more straightforward position for the man only need to locate the anus. The nerve endings found in the anus play a significant role in stimulating the woman relieving her duties in controlling their bodies.

Conclusion

The first step toward creating change in your life. Re-connecting with yourself, your partner and your place in the universal order, is the first step in a journey of one thousand miles. The destination is much less important than the journey. This is probably the most enduring theme of Kama Sutra. The quality of your journey is defined by your awareness of its beauty and the many details that make its progress delightful and joyful.

Our sexuality is something appealed to in our everyday lives. Our eyes are filled with titillation and provocation and this omnipresent, communal sexual expression may be at the root of our discontent. Everywhere we look, it's in our faces. Commodities and shrink-wrapped; sulfurized and bagged at the checkout counter, the banality of 21st Century sex penetrates us and desecrates the genuine spirituality, which is at the heart of human sexuality.

That spirituality at sexuality's heart is entirely love. Love is the nature of the universe. Wrought in the union of Shiva and Parvati and regulated in the fruit of their loins (which conquered evil, as we've read), love is reality itself. Love gives birth to compassion, the universal birthplace of all peace. When you love, you release energy into the universe, which multiples the love that is its nature. You feed the cosmic truth with your own and you participate in its health by becoming part of it. When this love is realized physically, the vibrational power of couples who love one another with an intentional and mindful sexuality becomes a powerful agent of goodness, illuminating the universe with an even brighter light than can possibly be imagined. That's why your sexuality exists and why it's so important. Sexuality is a spiritual commission to human beings. It's what we're born for – love not only felt but physically incarnated.

Living well and fully isn't something that just "happens". We can choose to let life roll over us and bob about in its currents like an errant cork, or we can choose to surf over its swells, governing ourselves as participants and not just bystanders. Being a bystander is easy. It's passive. But it's much less fun than actually being in the game. Those things that demand nothing of us have little reward save disappointment, and disappointment has no place in a life well lived.

Kama Sutra serves to remind us that sex, while a natural human activity, is as much an art form as life itself, also demanding active participation and understanding and the engagement of the whole person. That engagement is not only physical, or visceral. That engagement is intellectual and spiritual. The whole human being, when engaged, becomes a being of light, dancing in a limitless cosmos that not only needs but demands participation on a holistic level. It's not enough just to be. Being consciously, intentionally and mindfully engaged with our sexuality serves to hold together the universe by reinforcing the great love at its core. As once Shiva and Parvati's union saved the universe from the evil work of a demon, your union can be equally divine and equally salvific. This is a great and holy human commission that you can now begin to live out, joining with your partner as twin agents of the divine.

As a sexual being seeking a deeper and more fulfilling connection with your partner, you're also seeking a deeper and more fulfilling connection with the cosmos itself. Your part in the divine plan and in your divinely-gifted sexuality is part of what makes the universe an integrated whole. By learning to give sexuality the exalted and holy position in your life it deserves, you are becoming more attuned to what it means to be human. Approaching your sexuality as a reverent act of worship will not only bring you closer to the truth about yourself and your partner, it will bring you closer to the truth about the vast universe you live in and which your love helps to support the health of.

I thank you for reading this book. I hope and trust it will inform your life with your partner, bringing you both greater joy in every part of your lives together. I hope you come to enjoy the full and joyous incarnation of the deep connection that already exists between you. By re-igniting the flame of desire between you, you will draw closer to one another than you'd ever believed possible, even at the beginning of your relationship. Sexuality is a spiritual reality, not just a physical one. Acknowledging that truth and taking steps to live in it and glory in it is about to make your life a joyful journey of discovery and cosmic ecstasy.

May the spirit of the original cosmic lovers, Shiva and Parvati be with you on your journey. May your journey be one of unconditional and limitless love, after their example. May you know the joy of cosmic truth.

You are now ready to go off into the world of sexual exploration and have great orgasms from here on out. Stay curious and keep learning!

Printed in June 2023
by Rotomail Italia S.p.A., Vignate (MI) - Italy